EDUCATE, TRAIN AND TRANSFORM

**Toolkit on
Medical and Health
Professions Education**

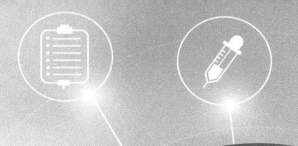

EDUCATE, TRAIN AND TRANSFORM

Toolkit on Medical and Health Professions Education

Editors

Dujeepa D. Samarasekera
Matthew C. E. Gwee

Centre for Medical Education (CenMED)
Yong Loo Lin School of Medicine
National University of Singapore

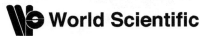

World Scientific

NEW JERSEY · LONDON · SINGAPORE · BEIJING · SHANGHAI · HONG KONG · TAIPEI · CHENNAI · TOKYO

Published by

World Scientific Publishing Co. Pte. Ltd.

5 Toh Tuck Link, Singapore 596224

USA office: 27 Warren Street, Suite 401-402, Hackensack, NJ 07601

UK office: 57 Shelton Street, Covent Garden, London WC2H 9HE

Library of Congress Cataloging-in-Publication Data

Names: Samarasekera, Dujeepa D., editor. | Gwee, Matthew C. E., editor.

Title: Educate, train and transform : toolkit on medical and health professions education /
editors, Dujeepa D. Samarasekera, Matthew C.E. Gwee.

Description: Hackensack, New Jersey : World Scientific, [2020] | Includes bibliographical references and index.

Identifiers: LCCN 2020001824 | ISBN 9789813279261 (hardback) | ISBN 9789813279278 (paperback) |
ISBN 9789813279285 (ebook) | ISBN 9789813279292 (ebook other)

Subjects: MESH: Education, Medical--organization & administration |
Education, Professional--trends | Health Personnel--education

Classification: LCC R737 | NLM W 18 | DDC 610.71/1--dc23

LC record available at https://lccn.loc.gov/2020001824

British Library Cataloguing-in-Publication Data

A catalogue record for this book is available from the British Library.

For any available supplementary material, please visit
https://www.worldscientific.com/worldscibooks/10.1142/11243#t=suppl

CONTENTS

ACKNOWLEDGEMENT

We would like to express our sincere gratitude to China Medical Board for providing the financial support.

We would also like to thank the Dean and colleagues from the Procurement Team of Finance, Yong Loo Lin School of Medicine, National University of Singapore as well as Office of Legal Affairs of National University of Singapore for your wholehearted support for this book.

We are grateful to have dedicated authors for the countless hours they have spent in writing the book section.

We would like to thank our colleagues from the Centre for Medical Education (CenMED), Yong Loo Lin School of Medicine, National University of Singapore for your assistance and constant support provided.

Lastly, we are grateful to have World Scientific Publishing Co. Pte Ltd for their support.

Editors

CONTRIBUTORS

W. David Carr PhD, ATC
Associate Professor, Department of Sports Medicine and Athletic Training, Missouri State University, United States of America

Zhi Xiong Chen BSc (Hons), MHPE, PhD
Assistant Dean (Education) and Senior Lecturer, Department of Physiology, Yong Loo Lin School of Medicine, National University of Singapore

Kirsty Forrest MBChB, BSc Hons, FRCA, FAcadMEd, MMEd, FANZCA
Professor & Dean of Medicine, Faculty of Health Sciences and Medicine, Bond University, Australia

Matthew C.E. Gwee BSc, PhD, MHPEd
Emeritus Professor & Chairman, International and Education Programmes, Centre for Medical Education, Yong Loo Lin School of Medicine, National University of Singapore, National University Health System, Singapore

Wayne Hazell MBBS, DipObs, GCCT, MClinED, FACEM
Associate Professor & Emergency Physician / Senior Medical Officer, University of Queensland (UQ) Northside Clinical Unit Site Co-Ordinator, Critical Care MD Program Site Co-Ordinator, Advanced Hospital Practice Semester Site Co-Ordinator, Faculty of Medicine, The University of Queensland, Australia

Marcus Alexander Henning CLTA, DipTch, BA, MA, MBus, PhD
Associate Professor, Centre for Medical and Health Sciences Education, University of Auckland, New Zealand

Paul Kneath Jones BSc, PGDip Advanced Practice
Honorary Associate Professor & Programme Director of Graduate Entry Medicine Programme, Swansea University School of Medicine, Swansea University, United Kingdom

Indika M. Karunathilake MBBS, MMedEd, FCGP, FCME, FHEA, FRCP (Edin)
Professor in Medical Education; Head, WHO Collaborating Centre for Medical Education; Faculty of Medicine, University of Colombo, Sri Lanka

Tang Ching Lau MBBS, M.MED (Int Med), MRCP (UK), FAMS, M.MED SC (Clin.Epid), FRCP (Edin), GDAcu (Singapore)
Vice-Dean (Education), Yong Loo Lin School of Medicine, National University of Singapore, National University Health System, Singapore; Senior Consultant, Division of Rheumatology, University Medicine Cluster, National University Health System, Singapore; Group Education Director, National University Health System, Singapore

Shuh Shing Lee BSc, M.Ed, PhD
Medical Educationalist, Centre for Medical Education, Yong Loo Lin School of Medicine, National University of Singapore, National University Health System, Singapore

Judy McKimm MBA, MA(Ed), BA(Hons), PGDip (HSW), CertEd, SFHEA, FAcadMed, FAMEE
Professor Emeritus of Medical Education, Swansea University Medical School, Swansea University, United Kingdom

Gominda G. Ponnamperuma MBBS, Dip. Psychology, MMEd, PhD
Professor, Department of Medical Education, Faculty of Medicine, University of Colombo, Sri Lanka

Gary D. Rogers MBBS, MGPPsych, PhD, FAMEE, FANZAHPE, PFHEA
Professor and Dean of the School of Medicine, Deakin University, Victoria, Australia

Dujeepa D. Samarasekera MBBS, MHPE, FAcadMEd, FAMS, FAMM, FAMEE, FRCP(Edin)
Senior Director, Centre for Medical Education (CenMED), Yong Loo Lin School of Medicine, National University of Singapore, National University Health System, Singapore; Director, Centre for Development of Teaching and Learning (CDTL), National University of Singapore, Singapore

Lambert Schuwirth MD, PhD
Professor of Medical Education, Director Prideaux Centre for Research in Health Professions Education, College of Medicine and Public Health, Flinders University, Adelaide, Australia; Professor for Innovative Assessment, Department of Educational Development and Research, Maastricht University, the Netherlands

Chay Hoon Tan MBBS, MMed (Psy), MMEd (Dundee), PhD
Visiting Consultant Psychiatrist, National University Hospital; Associate Professor, Department of Pharmacology, Yong Loo Lin School of Medicine, National University of Singapore, National University Health System, Singapore

FOREWORD

Educate, Train & Transform: Toolkit on Medical and Health Professions Education

I have always been a firm believer in treasuring and optimising every learning encounter with our students because we never know when one of these occasions will spark off an insight that may lead to a breakthrough on a personal or even global basis. It is important that everybody in the NUS Yong Loo Lin School of Medicine, from faculty to administrative staff, understands this early on. When I was asked to speak at my first Dean's Dialogue as Dean-Designate in 2018, I took the opportunity to set the expectation that, "in NUS Medicine, everyone teaches", and "the best teachers revolutionise learning". I continue to emphasise this point today, whether it be meeting a small group of Heads of Departments or addressing a full auditorium of administrative staff and directors.

The NUS Yong Loo Lin School of Medicine has come a long way in 115 years and has produced well over 10,000 medical and nursing professionals. It remains the top choice for students who wish to enter medical school in Singapore. In the coming years, our medical curriculum will be under tremendous pressure to evolve quickly as public expectations of healthcare increase. Doctors of the future will be treating Internet-savvy patients who expect quick, informed and convenient engagement with their doctors throughout their health journey.

This is 21st century healthcare.

With an anticipated overhaul of medical education in the horizon, teaching and maintaining a rigorous medical education curriculum must and should always remain our top priority as we continue to groom aspiring clinicians and scientists for Singapore.

Complacency has no place in our School. To remain Singapore's leading medical school, we need to continuously re-examine our curriculum delivery, and understand how we can keep pace with new learning methods that will retain our students' interest and allow us, as educators, to holistically assess them. The old methods of using textbooks to deliver facts is fast becoming obsolete as the growth of new knowledge outpaces traditional publication and accelerates the evolving practice of Medicine. As educators, we need to not only embrace lifelong learning but to evangelise it; this means learning new ways of teaching, figuring out how to evoke passion for Medicine in the Generation Z students, and teaching our students how to navigate doubts, evaluate evidence and explore new possibilities in Medicine.

Put together by the Centre for Medical Education and faculty members at the NUS Yong Loo Lin School of Medicine, **Educate, Train & Transform: Toolkit on Medical and Health Professions Education** serves as a guide for educators to refine their teaching methods and understand the psychology behind students' learning motivations. In seven chapters, this book details available tools and opportunities to spice up lesson delivery, incorporate frameworks to investigate, evaluate and support difficult learners. This book also helpfully touches on why training and preparation matters in building solid leadership. Ultimately, a robust management system makes a difference in the reformation of educational pedagogy in the face of changing health professional practice.

I trust that like-minded medical colleagues will find this book helpful, as they mentor younger colleagues and students in navigating the noble profession of Medicine.

I wish you a good read.

Chong Yap Seng MBBS, MMED, MRACOG, FAMS, MD
Lien Ying Chow Professor in Medicine
Dean, Yong Loo Lin School of Medicine
National University of Singapore

PREFACE

The *Educate, Train & Transform: Toolkit on Medical and Health Professions Education* was written to assist the new Biomedical Science and Clinician Educators to apply theoretical underpinnings to practical classroom and bedside teaching in an effective and meaningful way. The book's intent is to simplify theoretical concepts in a practical way for the educators involved in teaching-learning activities to effectively engage their learners as well as to develop programmes.

The book is divided into seven sections which cover aspects of health professional education. Each section starts with the practical scenario, common challenges faced by educators involved in medical and health professional training programmes. The chapters are divided into 'Why — the rationale, the theoretical underpinnings', 'What — the tools that can be used', and 'How — the Best Evidence Medical Education practices and approaches which could be applied in such a situation'.

Online edition will be available: https://www.worldscientific.com/worldscibooks/10.1142/11243

We are very grateful for all the authors of the chapters, the administrative staff at the Centre for Medical Education (CenMED) who assisted in developing this book, the leadership from the Yong Loo Lin School of Medicine, National University of Singapore for their encouragement and the publisher World Scientific Publishing Co. Pte Ltd. Last but not least, the China Medical Board for giving us the grant to make this book possible.

Editors:
Dujeepa D. Samarasekera & Matthew Gwee Choon Eng

LEARNING IN THE 21ST CENTURY — 'WHAT'S ALL THE FUSS ABOUT CHANGE?'

Indika M. Karunathilake and Dujeepa D. Samarasekera

Scenario

University *Serving with Heart*, ranked amongst one of the best medical schools in the region, and took pride in graduating the country's best practitioners every year for the last 100 years. Recently, the top leadership of the school announced that it will respond to the need to change to an integrated, technology-enhanced and student-centred curriculum. The news was greeted with much unhappiness amongst some faculty. Many felt there was no need to change since *Serving with Heart* had earned the status of a top-ranking school with high-performing graduates. The question was raised, 'So why should we change?'

Introduction

Medicine and Medical Education is in a continuous flux. Population growth, emergence of new diseases, and newer ways of managing patient conditions and the rapid changes to science and technology over the last few decades have transformed the way medicine is practiced. Accordingly, education and training of doctors and healthcare professionals has changed. This is further affected by factors such as exponential increase in medical knowledge in recent times, rapid changes to healthcare delivery, increased use of technology in the delivery of education and patient care. Higher expectations by students regarding the quality of education and by patients regarding the care they receive and changing attitudes regarding one's professional practice have contributed to the changes the way in which medicine should be taught and learned.[1]

Chapter 1: Why Change?

Changes in Medical Knowledge

'The burden we place on the medical student is far too heavy, and it takes some doing to keep from breaking his intellectual back'

Thomas Huxley, 1876

Medical/health professions education has traditionally been structured to progress from learning basic science in the early years to clinical training towards the latter part of the programme. This approach was mainly conceptualised following Flexner's report published in 1910.[2] However, recent advancements have greatly increased the quantum of scientific knowledge. The vast expansion of the horizons of medicine through science and technology no longer allows physicians and other health professionals to acquire all relevant knowledge to provide quality patient care. It is estimated that the existing medical knowledge doubles in every 5 years, outdating most of the knowledge gained during a 5-year medical program. In this context, simply adding more material or time to the curriculum will not be an effective strategy.[3]

Furthermore, changing disease patterns such as the increased disease burden from non-communicable diseases and emergence of virulent and newer infectious diseases mean that it is unreasonable to attempt to teach the entirety of medical knowledge during an undergraduate medical course. Thus, medical education has to continuously adapt with the changing learning and practice environments.[1]

'There remains gross overcrowding of most undergraduate curricula, acknowledged by teachers and deplored by students'.

General Medical Council, UK, 1993

Change in Healthcare Delivery

The health system is changing, with improved access to healthcare and more emphasis on the use of technology. The expansion of the private healthcare sector has both positive and negative implications. Changes in the disease burden result in a growing emphasis in health promotion and healthy lifestyles. A well-balanced health system is needed with community-based promotion and institution-based curative healthcare delivery to ensure a healthy society in the 21st century.[4]

Changes in Patients' Expectations

With the increasing availability and access to information, patients are well-informed about health and disease as well as the variety of options available for management. They no longer wish to be the passive recipients of medical opinion, but prefer to actively take part in the decision-making process. Therefore, doctors and health professionals need to be trained to adapt and practice in a positive manner aligned to the patient's needs.[1]

Patients and their families increasingly expect efficient, safe and cost-effective care from their medical professionals. Use of evidence-based medicine and employing current best practices in care management have become the cornerstone of contemporary clinical practice. There are many recent examples that show the society in general has become less tolerant of real or perceived deficiencies in healthcare delivery and, rather than being quiescent, has become increasingly litigious. Because of these reasons, it is important to develop curricula which encompasses current knowledge, best practices as well as developing students' cognitive and psycho-motor skills to adapt and adopt to dynamic practice conditions.

Changes in Doctors Themselves

Doctors too represent a cross section of the society. Their behaviour, attitudes, practices and aspirations are influenced by social, economic and political factors. Furthermore, we see health professionals placing more value on work-life balance, in order to mitigate the stressors of clinical practice. Their response to the above-mentioned changes could be very variable. These issues must be taken into consideration when we develop curricula and learning environments by providing good support structures and relevant inputs in ethics and professionalism.

Changes in Students

Students today come from a diverse social, ethnic and financial backgrounds and have attained high personal and academic achievements.

The sudden growth of medical schools both public and private sectors has also resulted in an increased need for trained medical teachers, with faculty positions falling vacant in many medical schools. Lack of effective government oversight or weak regulatory processes in many countries has led to poor standards.

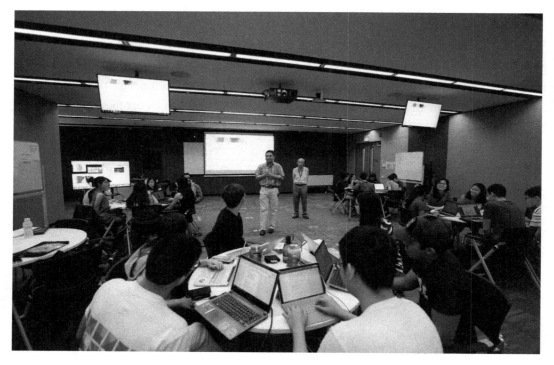

Medical students engaging in small group learning — Collaborative Learning Cases (CLC) at School of Medicine, National University of Singapore, Singapore Photo Credit: Yong Loo Lin School of Medicine, NUS.

Conclusion

This chapter highlights the rationale for change in the way we train medical students' and residents. Rapid changes in the practice environment and incorporating patient-centred care, enhanced through the use of technology are the main reasons for the reforms to the training programs.

Practice Highlights

- Practice of medicine has changed because of a rapid increase in population growth, emergence of new diseases, changes to management of disease conditions and advances to science and technology
- Medical education must also change to align with practice changes and to leverage on available contemporary best evidence in medical education
- The student profile and their expectations have changed
- There is increased use of technology in education
- Graduates are moving across practice settings and countries

Chapter 2: What to Change?

'Undertake something that is difficult, it will do you good. Unless you try to do something beyond what you have already mastered, you will never grow'.

— *Ronald E. Osborn*

Faculty Resistance to Change

One of the biggest challenges in education reform is when there is resistance from the faculty. Whilst the faculty continuously strive to foster a growth mindset in students, sometimes teachers themselves operate with a fixed mindset. This could be due to several factors as highlighted in the scenario at the beginning of this section. Faculty complacency is a key factor that could lead to resistance by teachers to curricular reform. Increasing pressures on staff with regard to clinical duties, teaching responsibilities and research commitments without adequate school level support or structures for career progression can be another critical factor. The best ways of changing faculty are to empower them by providing them the relevant knowledge and skill-sets through a contextually relevant faculty development program.[5]

Complexity of Medical Curriculum and Accountability

The Chapter 1 discussed the rapid changes taking place in medical education in order to align with the contemporary practice of medicine. This is mainly to assist and empower future doctors to provide quality care and be part of a technology driven multi-professional team.

With the advances in best evidence in medical education, most training curricula and assessment methods have become very complex.[6,7] It is inappropriate to continue to rely on outdated or ineffective methods of teaching. Innovative approaches are required to prepare doctors to practice in the new millennium. Use of best evidence practices in developing new medical curricula are known to decrease the volume of factual knowledge presented and to provide opportunities for choice. These focus on integrating the medical, social disciplines meaningfully, and for students to be practice ready in a hospital or community care setting. Special emphasis is given to developing skills and attitudes of students.[8,9] Traditional methods of teaching are not necessarily suitable for dealing with an expanding volume of material; indeed, it has been shown that students' learning styles deteriorate when they come into contact with the medical curriculum. Attempts to reduce the number of passive learning encounters, which encourages rote memorisation are not new. Studies have shown that students place little value on these passive activities as a method of learning, giving preference to active learning approaches such as learning by group discussions and through systematic exposure to future practice environments in small groups.[1] More specific examples will be provided in the subsequent sections in this book.

Curricular complexity can be managed by having a systematic and a structured governing process to ensure better oversight. This will also help generate data for continuously improving the quality of the learning environment by providing timely feedback regarding the program and faculty performance. These are vital areas to consider in the current context.

Information Technology in Medical Education

Medical education is rapidly changing and influenced by many factors including the changing healthcare environment, the changing role of the physician, altered societal expectations, rapidly changing medical science, and the diversity of pedagogical techniques.[10] Use of data analytics and artificial intelligence to improve learning and in the delivery of patient care will be the norm in the future. Unfortunately, very few medical curricula or training programs provide any exposure to students or residents in relevant information technology (IT) such as in programming or data analytics. Today's students will be practicing beyond the next 20 years and are expected and required to function effectively within ever-changing health systems.

Conclusion

Research in medical education has led to a better understanding of how students' learn.[11] Advanced approaches to education and new tools to aid learning have evolved and these will become the main themes of teaching medicine in the 21st century. Medical education has responded to the change in context of medical practice with far-reaching innovations. The need for change has been largely acknowledged and potential barriers have been identified.

Practice Highlights

- Resistance by faculty is a major change to curricular reforms. This needs to be addressed early and effectively
- In response to increased practice demands, medical curricula have become increasingly complex and good oversight is needed through a structured governance process
- Teaching-Learning and assessment formats must be based on best evidence practices
- Use of technology in education is key to enhance learning and development of both the students and faculty

Chapter 3: How to Change?

'It must be considered that there is nothing more difficult to carry out nor more doubtful of success nor more dangerous to handle than to initiate a new order of things'. Machiavelli, In 'The Prince' (1513).

The principal challenges in medical education can be categorised as changes occurring in the healthcare environment, the information explosion related to medicine and healthcare, and changes in the learner profile. Changes in the healthcare environment are driven by advances in technology, increasing costs, diversity of providers and settings, changing expectations of patients and the public (including professionalism, ethics and communication) and commodification of healthcare.

Two eminent medical educationists, Gale & Grant (1997) suggested that change is possible and practicable. They describe the change process in 10 steps.[12] Collins & Collins (2006) in their monograph for the Social Sector to accompany the famous book — *Good To Great* have also highlighted excellent practical insights to successfully engage a change process.[13] These are summarised below:

1. Establish the need for or the benefit of this change. It must be shared with all upon whom the change will have an impact. These include both the primary and secondary stakeholders such as the medical school faculty, students/parents, practitioners, patients/caregivers, the professional/regulatory bodies and the funders/sponsors. They must be involved from the very beginning, starting from the needs analysis if a change process is going to be successful. Consult widely with all those affected by the change.

2. Study and develop effective strategies to manage the powers who drive the school and the program so that the proposed reforms move forward, and the forces which might hinder it can be mitigated.

3. Design the innovation taking into account its feasibility, resources needed, an appropriate time scale and getting the right people on board.

4. Publicise the change widely, taking feedback with a view to amending the proposal. Once implemented modify the plans, redesigning the system in the light of experience.

5. Provide support in dealing with difficulties and maintaining change and evaluate the outcomes.

Information Explosion Related to Medicine and Healthcare

There is a global information explosion, which includes not only a rapid and exponential increase in published information, but also the short- and long-term effects of this growth.

The increasing quantum of knowledge in medicine no longer allows physicians to retain all knowledge that is necessary to provide quality patient care. Over 34,000 references are added to MEDLINE each month from approximately 4,000 journals, and the doubling time of medical knowledge is estimated to be approximately 5 years.[14] Knowledge is expanding faster than the ability to assimilate and apply it effectively; this is as true in education and patient care as it is in research.

Clearly, the simple inclusion of more material and/or time to the medical curriculum will not be an effective management strategy. Therefore, a fundamental change in the approach to medical education has become imperative. The importance of information technology as a tool for life-long learning and for accessing information has been realised.

Can we Use Affordable and Available Technology to Address and Prepare for Future Challenges in Medical Education?

There are many technologies currently used in medical education including simulation, E-learning/M-learning, virtual patients/virtual communities, virtual and augmented reality, artificial intelligence, and tools for sharing information and networking. Many of the features of these technologies can be implemented even within a resource poor setting because of the availability of free open source software and programmes.[15,16]

Simulation based and E-Learning to Change our Approach in Education to Face Future Challenges

Simulations are widely used for educational development. The aim of simulation is to imitate real patients, anatomic regions or clinical tasks, and mirror the real-life circumstances in which medical services are rendered. Simulations can fulfil a number of educational goals.[17,18]

E-learning and online learning can provide medical education with many affordable options. As an example, open source learning management system platforms such as MOODLE (modular object-oriented dynamic learning environment) are relatively low cost, yet used with high effectiveness in medical education. This technology can provide opportunities to change our approach in education to face future challenges. One example is the use of 'flipped classrooms' in which students review an online lecture before the face-to-face session, and come to the classroom to have an interactive session with the teacher.[19]

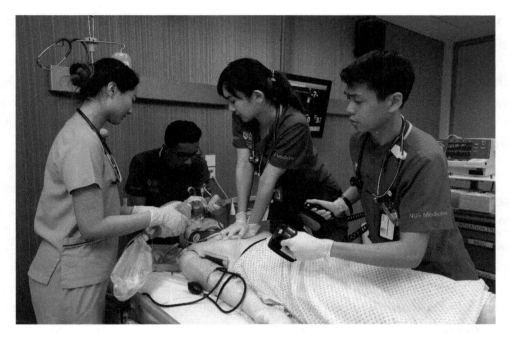

Medical and Nursing students engaging in simulation learning. Photo Credit: Yong Loo Lin School of Medicine, National University of Singapore, Singapore.

Virtual Reality for Medical Education

Virtual reality (VR) refers to the recreation of environments or objects as a complex, computer-generated image. In VR simulations, the computer display simulates the physical world and user interactions are with the computer within that simulated (virtual) world. Interaction can vary from looking around to interactively modifying the world. Augmented reality (AR) involves adding a virtual experience to information obtained from the real environment. Even though most virtual reality initiatives are very sophisticated and of high cost, availability of smart phones and affordable VR headsets, which can be purchased at low cost provide opportunities for implementing virtual learning.

Changes in the Learner Profile

It is important to note that changes in the learner profile lead to challenges as well. Present-day medical students are more technologically advanced than ever, and it is important for faculty to identify the inherent advantages as well as disadvantages faced by the 'digital natives' who make up the majority. These changes in the learner profile lead to different approaches to learning, presenting ongoing challenges to medical educators.

These challenges will become even more pronounced for countries and institutions with limited financial, human and infrastructural resources. It is perceived that technological advances that have led to many changes in health systems and medical education are beyond the reach of countries with limited resources even with the availability of open source material.[20]

Continuous Professional Development and the use of Online Learning

Providing continuous professional development (CPD) to faculty members and increasing numbers of health professionals working in diverse settings is a challenge for medical education.

The assumption held by many over the past several decades that the teachers involved in Health Professions Education programs are competent to teach once they specialise in their own subject areas and recruited as faculty is changing. Most medical schools and even accrediting agencies now mandate that faculty go through proper structured training as well as CPD. This will assist them to teach more effectively and enhance student learning.[21] Development of contextually relevant programs will ensure acquisition of necessary skills as well as the appropriate attitude to change the mindset of faculty towards curricular reforms.

Use of online platforms to provide real-time and convenient faculty development and CPS programs will yield higher returns for busy faculty members. There are many opportunities offered through online learning for CPD, driven by increasing access to the Internet and increasing availability of IT facilities, and facilities. The evidence base for online learning for CPD is gaining strength.[22,23] Access to information via the usage of repositories or digital libraries in medical education is on the rise. The Health Education Assets Library (HEAL) at http://www.healthcentral.org/ and the Multimedia Educational Resource for Learning and Online Teaching (MERLOT) at http://www.merlot.org/ are two examples for digital libraries. These are freely accessible resources of high-quality information that benefit medical educators and medical students alike.[24-26]

M-learning as an Opportunity for Continuous Professional Development

Mobile learning (M-Learning), offers many exciting opportunities for CPD. M-learning refers to learning via a mobile device such as a tablet or smartphone. Such devices are ubiquitous among doctors and offer an array of potential opportunities for CPD. M-Learning has progressed from e-mail and instant messaging services such as Yahoo, MSN, AOL and Skype, to more flexible and user friendly mobile applications such as WhatsApp and Viber for text, voice mode, video calling, as well as more sophisticated tools such as Articulate Studio for delivery of learning material and improvement of connectivity among learners in CPD.

Effectiveness of Technology Enhanced Medical Education in Postgraduate Medical Education

There is an ever-expanding body of evidence establishing the effectiveness of simulation in postgraduate medical education. Studies conducted worldwide within the postgraduate specialties of surgery, anaesthesiology, paediatrics and emergency medicine have demonstrated that simulation is effective in teaching patient safety and practical procedures, leading to better adherence to safety guidelines and improved clinical practice. Several studies have demonstrated that VR simulators can effectively discriminate novices from experts and that VR-trained residents in surgery performed better on time taken to complete procedures and overall operating room performance when compared with those who were traditionally trained.[27]

Inculcating and Enhancing Values

Even though technology and science will radically transform medical education and the practice of medicine in the future, what will remain unchanged is the relationship between the health professional the patient. Building trust with the patient as well as with other members of the team will be a central core of effective clinical practice. Enhancing the trainees' values and skills such as communication skills, attitudinal attributes and ethical practice are essential to prepare them for teamwork and the role of evidence-based practice. These core tenets should all find a place in a revised curriculum for young health professionals to develop effective relationships with patients and in developing a multi-professional team approach to healthcare delivery.

These innovative approaches to learning require appropriate assessment strategies. Subsequent sections and chapters will discuss more details regarding the development of contemporary best evidence assessment strategies such as programmatic assessment and tools such as Objective Structured Clinical Examination (OSCE).[28,29]

Conclusion

Curricular reform and change management require systematic and evidence-based planning and execution. However, sustaining the changes and the change process requires improvement of the faculty skill-sets through structured faculty development programs aligned to institutional incentive structures. Curricular reforms and changes must enhance and build trust between the institution and faculty and with our graduates, as well as patients. Technology is an enabler and the appropriate use offers many opportunities to overcome challenges discussed in medical education.

Practice Highlights

- A systematic and structured approach must be taken to manage curricular reform based on the best evidence in medical education
- Incorporating learning methods to promote active learning and the use of technology platforms to drive millennial learners is important in the current context
- Developing the skills-set of faculty through appropriate faculty development and CPD programs is necessary to ensure that reforms are sustainable and progressive
- Inculcating values among students and building trust with key stakeholders will remain the core of change management

References

1. Schuwirth LWT, van der Vleuten CPM. Challenges for educationalists. *BMJ*. 2006;333(7567): 544–6.

2. Irby DM, Cooke M, O'Brien BC. Calls for reform of medical education by the Carnegie Foundation for the Advancement of Teaching: 1910 and 2010. *Academic Medicine*. 2010;85(2):220–7.

3. Samarasekera DD, Goh PS, Lee SS, Gwee MCE. The clarion call for a third wave in medical education to optimise healthcare in the twenty-first century. *Medical Teacher*. 2018;40(10):982–5.

4. Karunathilake IM. Health changes in Sri Lanka: Benefits of primary health care and public health. *Asia Pacific Journal of Public Health*. 2012;24(4):663–71.

5. Lee SS, Dong C, Yeo SP, Gwee MC, Samarasekera DD. Impact of faculty development programs for positive behavioural changes among teachers: A case study. *Korean Journal of Medical Education*. 2018;30(1):11–22.

6. Harden RM, Grant J, Buckley G, Hart IR. BEME Guide No. 1: Best evidence medical education. *Medical Teacher*. 1999;21(6):553–62.

7. Densen P. Challenges and opportunities facing medical education. *Transactions of American Clinical and Climatological Association*. 2011;122:48–58.

8. Quintero GA. Medical education and the healthcare system — Why does the curriculum need to be reformed? *BMC Medicine*. 2014;12(1):213.

9. *Innovative Models of Medical Education in the United States Today: An Overview with Implications for Curriculum and Program Evaluation*. Washington, DC: National Academies Press 1983.

10. Khay Guan Y. The future of medical education. *Singapore Medical Journal.* 2019;60(1):3–8.

11. *How people learn II: Learners, Contexts, and Cultures.* Washington, DC: National Academies Press 2018.

12. Gale R, Grant J. AMEE Medical Education Guide No. 10: Managing change in a medical context: Guidelines for action. *Medical Teacher.* 1997;19(4):239–49.

13. Collins JC, Collins, J. *Good to Great and The Social Sectors: A Monograph to Accompany Good to Great: Random House Business.* 2006. 48 p.

14. Karunathilake I. Technology enhanced learning with limited resources — transforming limitations into advantages. *South East Asian Journal of Medical Education.* 2017;11.

15. Ranasinghe P, Wickramasinghe SA, Pieris WAR, Karunathilake I, Constantine GR. Computer literacy among first year medical students in a developing country: A cross sectional study. *BMC Research Notes.* 2012;5(1):504.

16. Yapa, YMMM, Dilan MMNS, Karunaratne, WCD, Widisinghe,CC, Hewapathirana, R. Karunathilake IM. Computer literacy & attitudes towards e-learning among Sri Lankan Medical Students. *Sri Lanka Journal of Bio-medical Informatics.* 2012;3:83–97.

17. Beetham H, Sharpe R. *Rethinking Pedagogy for a Digital Age: Designing for 21st Century Learning;* 2013.

18. Masters K, Ellaway RH, Topps D, Archibald D, Hogue RJ. Mobile technologies in medical education: AMEE Guide No. 105. *Medical Teacher.* 2016;38(6):537–49.

19. Moffett J. Twelve tips for "flipping" the classroom. *Medical Teacher.* 2015;37(4):331–6.

20. Kimble C. The Impact of Technology on Learning: Making Sense of the Research. *Policy Brief.* Aurora, CO.: Mid-Continent Regional Educational Lab; 1999.

21. Samarasekera DD, Lee SS, Findyartini A, Mustika R, Nishigori H, Kimura S, *et al.* Faculty development in medical education: An environmental scan in countries within the Asia pacific region. *Korean Journal of Medical Education.* 2020;32(2):119–30.

22. Phillips JL, Heneka N, Bhattarai P, Fraser C, Shaw T. Effectiveness of the spaced education pedagogy for clinicians' continuing professional development: A systematic review. *Medical Education.* 2019;53(9):886–902.

23. Shaw T, Barnet S, McGregor D, Avery J. Using the Knowledge, Process, Practice (KPP) model for driving the design and development of online postgraduate medical education. *Medical Teacher.* 2015;37(1):53–8.

24. Pathirana TI, Palagama S, Nazeer I, Karunathilake, IM. Developing an online CPD module on management of breast cancer for general practitioners in Sri Lanka — A need analysis. *South East Asian Journal of Medical Education.* 2015;9(1):58–61.

25. Kulatunga GG, Marasinghe RB, Karunathilake IM, Dissanayake VH. Development and implementation of a web-based continuing professional development (CPD) programme on medical genetics. *Journal of Telemedicine and Telecare.* 2013;19(7):388–92.

26. Kulatunga GG, Marasingha RB, Karunathilake IM, Dissanayake VHW. Introduction of web based continuous professional development to Sri Lanka. *Sri Lanka Journal of Bio-medical Informatics.* 2013;3:127.

27. Seymour NE, Gallagher AG, Roman SA, O'Brien MK, Bansal VK, Andersen DK, & Satava RM. Virtual reality training improves operating room performance: results of a randomized, double-blinded study. *Annals of Surgery*. 2002; 236(4): 458–464. https://doi.org/10.1097/00000658-200210000-00008

28. Hodges B, Turnbull J, Cohen R, Bienenstock A, Norman G. Evaluating communication skills in the objective structured clinical examination format: Reliability and generalizability. *Medical Education*. 1996;30(1):38–43.

29. Schuwirth LW, Van der Vleuten CP. Programmatic assessment: From assessment of learning to assessment for learning. *Medical Teacher*. 2011;33(6):478–85.

CURRICULUM ORGANISATION 'WHY CAN'T I JUST TEACH WHAT I KNOW?'

Dujeepa D. Samarasekera, Zhi Xiong Chen, Matthew C.E. Gwee

Scenario

Associate Professor Ashvin from the Department of Surgery and Assistant Professor Ben from the Department of Biochemistry were lamenting over the need to align their teaching outcomes to that specified by their institution's curriculum committee. They were upset that their students would no longer be able to benefit from their expertise this way, because they could no longer teach the way they had been taught many years ago. Since Associate Professor Ashvin and Assistant Professor Ben would no longer be able to deliver the curricular content they were comfortable with, they were considering getting the syllabi from their friends in other institutions and delivering it to their students.

Introduction

Effective and efficient curriculum organisation has become one of the major focus of medical and health professional schools recently. This is due to its direct impact on the delivery of quality healthcare by practitioners. Medical and Health Professional education have more recently learned best practices in curriculum development due to extensive research done as well as gathering of medical school data relating to effective designs. The key challenge in adapting the best evidence to design and implement curricula across the globe is the reluctance of faculty to change. This may be due to several reasons. Lack of understanding of contemporary best evidence practices in curricular design; resource limitations; larger student cohorts with fewer faculty; increased administrative burden due to the demands of quality assurance and accreditation agencies; and institutional demands for the faculty to engage extensively in research as well as in the provision of professional services are major contributory factors. The section will explore some of these critical areas and share contemporary practices based on Best Evidence Medical Education, i.e. BEME, in developing and organising a curriculum for health professions education.

Chapter 1: Why Is It Important to Contextualise Learning?

Before we begin to dissect the scenario, it is important to ask the question: "Do Ashvin and Ben indeed share the same learning outcomes as the institution but with misaligned content?" or 'Do Ashvin and Ben have content that fit their own learning outcomes, which are nonetheless, misaligned from those of the institution?' It would seem like the latter.

Several questions need to be asked. Why is it important for the institution to develop her own curriculum? Why is it important for learning outcomes to be aligned among all the educators of the institution? What are the possible reasons for Ashvin's and Ben's negative reactions and resistance? Is it appropriate for Ashvin and Ben to adopt syllabi 'wholesale' from other institutions for their own teaching purposes? If not, what are the concerns and pitfalls regarding this? How do we overcome this 'adoption' mentality and what is the right way to go about it? To what extent should a 'foreign' curriculum be adopted? Through exploring these questions and more, we will obtain a better understanding of 'curriculum organisation'.

First of All, What is a Curriculum?

It is useful to begin our discussion on 'curriculum organisation' by asking the important question 'what is a curriculum?'. We can then proceed to discuss several aspects of a curriculum specially designed for medical and health professions education in the 21st century.

'Most human learning does not occur by design. The classroom is unique because it is a designed educational experience'.[1]

A curriculum is essentially an educational blueprint specially designed for formal student learning to achieve a specific set of outcomes. Not only does a curriculum document the educational activities intended for student learning, but it also provides students (i.e. the learners) with the learning experience they will need and will receive when undergoing a prescribed course (programme) of study. For students undergoing a medical or an allied health professional course, the learning experience is further enhanced and enriched at specially dedicated 'classrooms', i.e. at various clinical sites (which are also often engaged in service provision), in which opportunities abound for students to also learn from their clinical teachers, as well as patients.

Thus, a curriculum is an educational blueprint that informs students of the educational experience they can expect to receive when undergoing a given course of study as well as for the teachers or educators to develop those learning experiences. A curriculum, therefore, serves to document the key educational elements systematically organised (or designed) to inform students of the total educational experience intended for their effective learning in a given course (or programme) of study.

Thus, a curriculum needs to specify:

- What course content should students learn? (not what Ashvin or Ben prefers to teach or 'import' to teach)
- How should students learn the course content, i.e. how should the course content be delivered to students as instruction for their learning in order to acquire the intended learning outcomes prescribed for the course — Knowledge, Skills and Attitudes — in the learning domains? (not how Ashvin or Ben *thinks* or *feels* the course should be taught)
- How should students be assessed (or tested) on their acquisition of adequate, appropriate and relevant learning outcomes, i.e. how should students provide valid and reliable evidence on their acquisition of relevant:
  - (i) Knowledge (i.e. the factual course content) and associated intellectual skills in the cognitive (or knowledge) domain of learning (in simple terms the 'knowing' domain of learning)? (knowledge that students actually need to know and not what Ashvin or Ben *thinks* or *feels* they need to know)
  - (ii) Skills in the psychomotor skills domain (i.e. the 'doing' domain)? (skills that students actually need to know and not what Ashvin or Ben *thinks* or *feels* they need to know)
  - (iii) Attitudes (as reflected in the behaviour patterns of an individual such as an individual's interpersonal skills, i.e. the 'soft skills' or 'EQ' of an individual in the attitudes or affective ('feeling') domain? (attitudes that students actually need to acquire and not only the transference of Ashvin's or Ben's individual personality or those suggested by the 'adopted' syllabi to students)
- Any other educational experience specially and systematically organised for students in the course (programme) of study.

Thus, a curriculum is essentially a learning system designed for a given course of study and is, therefore, a specially planned learning experience for students (Fig. 1).

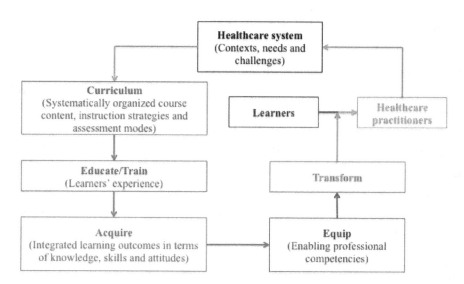

Fig. 1. The stages that transform today's students to become tomorrow's competent healthcare practitioners are based on systematically organising key educational elements (course content, modes of instruction and assessment) into a curriculum, which documents the total student learning experience required to achieve the intended outcomes of learning in a given course (or programme) of study.

'*The central mission of medical education is to improve the quality of healthcare delivered by doctors: what doctors do, and how and when they do it depends on the quality of medical education. We must get it right*'.[2]

Any educational curriculum specially designed for a medical or health profession course in the 21st century must ensure that education can serve the needs of healthcare practice; after all, education and practice are two interdependent sub-systems within the overall healthcare system.[2] Moreover, the educational experience specially designed for the students as they undergo their learning journey through their respective courses must ensure that the curriculum will provide the intended learning experience to educate, train and transform today's students to become tomorrow's competent healthcare practitioners who are fit to deliver healthcare that can meet the needs, demands and challenges of patients and the community in the 21st century. Ultimately, the end-products of education will be the new generation of competent healthcare practitioners upon their graduation.

Therefore, it is likely that the learning outcomes of Ashvin's and Ben's lessons do not sufficiently serve the needs of healthcare practice, and that the educational experience that leads to the current learning outcomes may not be relevant for producing competent healthcare practitioners. Hence, there is a need for the institution to lay down the curriculum and establish the learning outcomes for educators to align and adapt. It should be a curriculum that is driven by the need to produce healthcare practitioners who are fully adept to meet the needs of the local context while acknowledging the constraints and exploiting the strengths of the local education environment. The converse is a curriculum that is pulled in all directions and fragmented by various 'agents of interests' and sociocultural nuances exhibited by the learners and educators — a case of the 'tail wagging the dog'. So, what are the tools and opportunities available for developing a curriculum for contextualised learning instead of simply 'importing and adopting' syllabi from other institutions?

Practice Highlights

- Learning must be contextualised through a curriculum that is informed by the contexts, needs and challenges of the healthcare system.
- The curriculum in terms of the knowledge, skills and attitudes that it delivers to the learners should be constantly shaped by the healthcare system that it serves through a feedback loop.
- In turn, this will affect the content to be delivered, instructional strategies to be adopted and assessment modes to be undertaken.

Chapter 2: What Are the Tools And Opportunities Available?

In order to develop a coherent curriculum that will deliver the desired learning outcomes and eventually produce competent healthcare practitioners fit for 21st-century practice, it is important for the curriculum to be underpinned by a sound educational framework or model during the development phase. At the same time, curriculum developers would need to be attuned to current constraints, challenges and contexts to turn them into opportunities to develop a contextualised curriculum.

The SPICES Curriculum Model

In more recent years, several disruptive forces have made it imperative for education and practice to undertake major changes in order to optimise health outcomes in healthcare. Thus, special attention will be required in designing a curriculum for undergraduate students in medical and health professions courses in the 21st century. Several significant educational paradigm shifts must be incorporated into the curriculum to ensure that the end-products of education are students who upon graduation will become the new generation of competent healthcare practitioners who have the capability to optimise 'health benefits' for their patients in the 21st century.

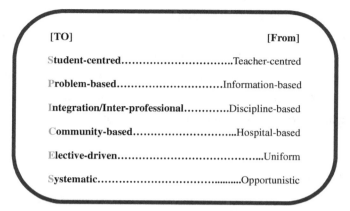

Fig. 2. Key features of the SPICES Curriculum Model. Each feature (category) in the model should be read from right to left to determine the stage reached (or the stage intended to be reached) by an institution at a given time point.

The SPICES Curriculum Model proposed by Harden, Snowden and Dunn in 1984[3] incorporates many of the key features required for the design of a 21st-century curriculum for undergraduate students in medical and health professions education. Each key feature (or category) is represented as a continuum along a horizontal line to accommodate and reflect the realistic differences achieved in each category by different institutions at different time points (Fig. 2).

How Do the Key Features In the SPICES Curriculum Model Support the Design of a Curriculum For Medical and Health Professions Education In the 21st Century?

The students who undergo medical and health professions education today will need to undergo the process of transformation through transformative learning to become competent healthcare practitioners in the future.[4]

'*We regard transformative learning as the highest of three successive levels, moving from informative to formative to transformative learning. … Transformative learning is the proposed outcome of instructional reforms*'.[4]

Generally, many of the key features proposed in the SPICES Curriculum Model represent key transformative processes that will support the change in status from students to practitioners as follows:

- Student-centred Learning (ScL)

Traditionally (especially in the 20th and early 21st century), student learning strongly focused on the passive teaching of factual course content delivered by the teacher using, predominantly, didactic lectures in which students simply 'sit, listen, and take and take notes … and then, memorize, recall and regurgitate in exams'.

Today, ScL is strongly advocated and recommended, mainly because it will involve the active participation of students in the teaching–learning process. In such a learning environment, students are more likely to develop greater responsibility and ownership for their own learning, thus becoming self-directed learners. In doing so, they are also more likely to embark on continuous lifelong learning that is self-driven and self-motivated based on self-assessed needs from time to time, which is so critical for maintaining their currency in practice.

- Problem-based

Today, student learning in healthcare education is aimed at not only what, but also how students should learn. If the focus is mainly on what to learn, then it is likely that students will progressively develop habits of memorising factual course content and, thus, engage in rote-learning, i.e. superficial learning with little understanding of the subject matter.[5]

However, if student learning is also focused on how the students learn, then a problem-based approach for student learning can be expected to progressively develop the ability of students to analyse, integrate, evaluate and apply knowledge and information to educational problems posed. Such regular practice in problem-solving will facilitate the development of intellectual skills such as critical thinking and reasoning, which can in turn augment the ability of students to solve problems and make good decisions with sound judgment as future healthcare practitioners.

- Integration/Inter-professional

Traditionally, the undergraduate medical curriculum was highly discipline-specific — clearly exemplified by the 'great divide' between the preclinical and clinical phases of medical education. Then, there was little 'crosstalk' among the disciplines, especially between the preclinical and clinical phases! Instead, each had a vested interest in guarding its own discipline, and 'silos' (little disciplinary kingdoms) prevailed.

'*Each department is responsible for some part of the education of a medical student, but no department should forget that it is no more than a part of the whole which is responsible for the education of the whole student and the fulfilment of the overall objective*.'[6]

Today, there is greater realisation that every discipline must lend its weight to the curriculum in a coherent and meaningful way whereby the overall outcome is greater than the sum of its parts. Every discipline must contribute its educational 'building block', which collectively will equip and transform students to become competent practitioners.[6] The medical curriculum must, therefore, aim at closer integration of its diverse disciplines instead of designing a discipline-centric curriculum in which student learning is compartmentalised, i.e. discipline-specific. After all, healthcare is practiced in an integrated fashion within the health system and there is no reason why the healthcare education should not reflect this!

'In [the delivery of] health care, patients have long depended on the grit of individual doctors and nurses. But in modern medicine, providing superior care has become so complex that no lone practitioner, no matter how driven, can do it all. Today great [patient] care requires great collaboration– gritty teams of clinicians who all relentlessly push for improvement'.[7]

Inter-professional education is now strongly advocated for undergraduates in medical and other health professions education in order to facilitate the development of collaborative habits for their respective future roles.[7] This will help to transform the students into practitioners who are more prepared to collaborate, not only inter-professionally, but also with patients under their care and consequently optimise health outcomes for patients. Such a mindset change would require changes in habit, attitude and behaviour, which can only come about through regular 'practice of integration' that is intentionally and purposefully built into the curriculum.

- Community-based

Today, the clinical learning experience of medical students should not be confined to the hospital setting only. Students should also be given every opportunity to learn from a community-based setting. This will transform and educationally prepare the students to take on future roles such as primary care physicians, a likely trend in the 21st century.

In Community Based Medical Education (CBME) learners, clinical training is simulated in a community setting exposing them to patients being managed in their own homes, ambulatory community clinics and other similar social settings.

With increasing aging populations, falling birth rates and increasing lifespans coupled with decreasing 'health spans' especially in developed nations, there are more to take care with less; patients will require integrated care that demands an in-depth understanding of community settings and challenges in order to intervene and manage in ways that will provide patients with the best chance for recovery, healing and re-integration into society.

- Elective-driven

In the past, there was little room for flexibility that will allow students to learn beyond what was prescribed in the standard curriculum. Such an approach assumed every student had the same interest and, even if not, could be shoe-boxed into having the same interest. Such a one-size-fits-all approach resulted in the mass production of undifferentiated healthcare practitioners who may not be fully motivated to do what they were supposed to do or equipped to deal with the diverse nature of healthcare challenges presented.

In the SPICES Curriculum Model, the need to grow a community of motivated healthcare practitioners with diverse strengths and skillsets is recognised. This is achieved through the provision of electives that focus on specific areas such as medical education or clinical research, for students to select based on their interests and motivation. This will result in a pool of healthcare practitioners who are motivated, prepared and equipped to tackle different dimensions of healthcare in an integrated manner.

- Systematic

Traditionally, medical students acquired knowledge and skills through an apprenticeship-based approach that relies on being attached to a 'master' clinician with learning often taking place in an opportunistic and unstructured fashion. In the SPICE Curriculum Model, this is overcome by having students learn through acquiring experiences in a structured program that takes them systematically from one point to another, connecting the points along the learning continuum, scaffolding and reinforcing their learning along the way. This is in stark contrast to the random, illogical and often quantum leaps that students have to go through during their 'scattered and irregular-paced' learning under the apprenticeship model whereby the learning experience is greatly variable and highly dependent on individual mentors.

Therefore, it is important for Ashwin and Ben to consider whether their lessons contain these elements of the SPICES Curriculum Model, and not simply 'import' syllabi from other institutions. If it does not; why not and how can they adapt their lessons to incorporate these elements? If these elements are present, how can each element be improved upon and is there any missing element?

What are the other opportunities available for a curriculum to be developed and evaluated, and to ensure quality?

Disruptive Forces As Opportunities of Change

Technology as a key player

'Technology has begun to transform social class, economic activity, political discourse, working life, and the limits of human activity'.[8]

'Artificial intelligence will reshape the world in ways we can't imagine, much as the Internet and the printing press did at their inceptions'.[9]

We now live in changing times. In particular, we now live in the era of the Internet, i.e. era of the super information highway! Today, at the click of a button, we can obtain a galore of information appearing before our very eyes in just a few seconds: attractive text, colourful graphics, stunning pictures and even live video streaming. Such is the power of the Internet, which has also heralded the advent of technology that now strongly impacts not only our daily lives, but also the education and practice of healthcare delivery. Technology is now considered a key disruptive force of change for education and healthcare practice![10] This further underscores the interdependence of the two sub-systems, education and practice, within the overall healthcare delivery system.

Other disruptive forces of change

All disruptive forces of change have the potential to improve healthcare practice. This, in turn, presents opportunities for educational change in order to provide the most relevant and up-to-date learning for students that will prepare them for the most current situation today and tomorrow. Such disruptive forces must, therefore, be taken into consideration by curriculum developers–designers in order to optimise the development and design of a curriculum. Some of these disruptive forces are advances made in medical domains in terms of knowledge, science and technology, e.g. wearable biosensors and incorporation of Artificial Intelligence (AI) in providing optimal care to patients. Use of big data and data analytics to personalise treatment as well as to predict illnesses of individuals and groups. Furthermore, greater focus on patient-centred care, team care of patients and patient-safety in order to optimise health outcomes for patients. Lee and Duckworth[7] have clearly expressed that '... *in modern medicine, providing superior care has become so complex that no lone practitioner, no matter how driven, can do it all. Today, great care requires great collaboration...'*

Because of this, Ashvin and Ben cannot go on to '*just teach what they know*' because '*what they know*' may be neither sufficient nor relevant for what students need to know in order to deal with the disruption to healthcare practice brought about by technological advances and sociocultural changes. Instead, Ashvin and Ben could turn these uncomfortable disruptions into opportunities that can contribute to a reformed curriculum that is constantly informed, contextualised and relevant. 'Importing' syllabi from other institutions may not be able to address or be adequate in harnessing these disruptive forces of change as opportunities, since these 'syllabi' may be developed for and cater to the unique contexts, needs and challenges of other healthcare systems and settings.

A curriculum is dynamic and never static. A curriculum has been defined by some experts as '...*activities provided for the students by the school... ...[suggesting] a rather static collection of learning experiences... But in reality, [a] curriculum is much more: it is dynamic, not static... ...it varies with its participants... ...it changes in subtle ways even when it is apparently unchanging. In short, it has an existence which goes beyond the concept of a static listing or description of its formal components. Indeed, participants in a curriculum — teachers and learners — tend to endow their curriculum with a 'life' of its own when they refer to it or to its components'.*[11]

A Dynamic Curriculum Needs to Be Critically Reviewed Regularly

A curriculum is, therefore, a dynamic entity and has a 'life' of its own.[11] It must, therefore, be reviewed regularly to determine whether or not the curriculum is still relevant, i.e. whether or not it is still adequate and appropriate for its intended educational purpose. However, over the course of time, disruptive forces, including changing trends, issues, priorities and strategies in education, will make it imperative for educators to undertake a curriculum review. Any aspect of a curriculum found 'lacking', i.e. inadequate and/or inappropriate, must be promptly updated, i.e. promptly revised or refined!

The regular review and updation of a curriculum to overcome any shortcoming or deficiency are deemed to be highly critical especially in the education of medical and health profession students. Failure to do so can result in, firstly, the onset of 'diseases of the curriculum' such as 'Curriculosclerosis' described as *'By far the most crippling disease, and tragically also one of the most prevalent... ...[It has been defined as a] 'hardening of the categories'... ... an extreme form of departmentalization... ...that becomes a stifling, inhibiting influence on normal development and function of the curriculum... In its most extreme disease state, this departmentalization manifests itself in a kind of social territoriality... ...a vested interest... ... [to establish dominance] on the importance of the department [in terms of hours allocated to teaching of the discipline]... Design of the curriculum can then seem to be more of a power struggle than an educational-planning venture'.*[11]

Several other 'diseases' have also been described including *'Carcinoma of the Curriculum, Curriculoarthritis, Curriculum Disesthesia, Iatrogenic Curriculitis, Curriculum Hypertrophy, Idiopathic Curriculitis, Intercurrent Curriculitis, Curriculum Ossification'.*[11]

Another serious and major outcome of an obsolete curriculum is the production of 'ill-equipped graduates' at the end of the course — a serious concern that is well documented in The Lancet Global Independent Commission Report (Health Professionals For A New Century: Transforming Education To Strengthen Health Systems In An Interdependent World), which clearly expressed that *'Professional education has not kept pace with these challenges, largely because of fragmented, outdated, and static curricula that produce ill-equipped graduates'.* The Report has also emphasised that *'...ineffective 20th century educational strategies are unfit to tackle 21st century challenges'.*[4]

Similar sentiments have also been expressed by the Executive Vice-President and CEO of the American Medical Association (AMA) in the foreword of the book 'Health Systems Science' published by the AMA Education Consortium.

'Medical school curricula focus and overall structure remain stubbornly captives of early twentieth-century thinking. The result is an ever-widening gap between how physicians in the United States are trained and educated and the realities of the modern health care environment'.[12]

Hence, it is important for Ashvin and Ben to review their lessons' content materials, instructional strategies and assessment modes, to be in line with the overall curriculum review, and to remain compatible with a dynamic curriculum.

Practice Highlights

- The SPICES Curriculum Model is a framework for developing a curriculum that is student-centric, tackles real-world problems, integrates with other professions, community-focused, promotes diverse learning through electives and systematic.
- Disruptive forces should be viewed as opportunities to review, redevelop and re-evaluate the relevance and quality of a curriculum.
- A dynamic curriculum needs to be constantly reviewed and 'kept on its toes'.

Chapter 3: How Can These Be Applied in a Coherent Strategy?

Harnessing a curriculum framework, technology and other opportunities arising from disruptive forces of change, we ask the question how can all these be applied to design and develop a curriculum that is engaging for 21st-century learners, adoptable by 20th-century teachers and remain relevant for 22nd-century healthcare practice. What sort of strategy should we take and what do we need to consider? But perhaps before we address these questions, we should first ask what is the primary goal of a curriculum for today's medical and health profession courses?

As discussed earlier, a curriculum is essentially a learning system design, i.e. an educational blueprint, consisting of 'key educational elements' systematically organised into a given course (or programme) of study. Thus, the 'key educational elements' will document, not only the educational experience of students (the learners) undergoing the course, but also stipulate the intended learning outcomes, i.e. the knowledge, skills and attitudes, that students need to acquire in a given discipline.

Thus, the primary goal of a curriculum for such professional courses in the 21st century is to ensure that the educational experience of students will determine (through the assessment strategies) the expected outcomes acquired by students in their learning, i.e. the professional competencies acquired, at the end of a given course of study. In this context then, the educational experience of students is expected to result in the transformation of today's students into tomorrow's competent healthcare practitioners who are fit to deliver healthcare that can meet the needs, demands and challenges of patients and the community in the 21st century.

The transformative 'key educational elements' in a curriculum for such professional courses in the 21st century will, therefore, include:

- Specific content for each discipline in a given course of study, i.e. the diverse educational 'building blocks' that students first need to acquire from each discipline, which will collectively equip them with enabling new professional competencies required for transforming the students into competent healthcare practitioners.
- Instructional strategies used for delivery of the content for students to acquire the educational 'building blocks', i.e. the intended learning outcomes arising from the knowledge, skills and attitudes associated with each discipline in the course.
- Closely aligned assessment modes to assess students' acquisition of relevant, i.e. adequate and appropriate, learning outcomes; in other words, students need to provide valid and reliable evidence of relevant acquisition of the intended learning outcomes acquired in the course of their learning.

These are three elements that Ashvin and Ben need to consider when refreshing and transforming their lessons in order to align them to the overall curriculum. Teaching and assessing the same thing in the same way may not be ideal, and these elements may not be optimal in syllabi that are 'imported and adopted' from other institutions.

The Close Relationship Between Education and Practice: Implications For the Development and Design of a Curriculum

The education and training programme of students in an undergraduate medical or allied health profession course is intended to transform today's students into tomorrow's competent healthcare practitioners. The curriculum, i.e. the educational programme, for these students must, therefore, incorporate transformative learning strategies in order to ensure the transformation of these students into competent healthcare practitioners. Therefore, there is a need to ensure the relevance of the curriculum to their future practice.[2]

Thus, a curriculum for students in the medical and health professions courses must be developed and designed on the basis of the close link and the interdependence between education and practice within the healthcare delivery system, i.e. the curriculum must ensure that it is closely aligned to the needs of healthcare practice. Only then can healthcare educators be able to optimise the development and design of a curriculum for students in these courses.

As mentioned earlier, changing trends, issues, priorities and strategies over time are likely events that may necessitate a review of the curriculum. This is because such events that usually arise from the disruptive forces of change are usually expected to strongly impact healthcare practice. Hence, it is crucial that education practice is nimble, current and responsive enough to develop and design a curriculum to match the ever-changing needs of healthcare practice without compromising core values.

Unless Ashvin and Ben have been using yesterday's healthcare practice to meet today's healthcare needs and challenges, they should not assume the same education practice and content to be relevant or sufficient to develop future healthcare practitioners who would be in charge of caring for their health tomorrow. Syllabi from other institutions may also not be entirely suitable as they may not be fully contextualised to the settings of the healthcare system that future healthcare practitioners are supposed to carry out their practice. At this can produce learners who do not fully understand the challenges and needs of the healthcare system that they will one day operate in, and transform them into healthcare practitioners who are not prepared socioculturally to serve the local patient community.

The Need To Develop Cultural Sensitivity In a Globalised World

We also now live in a 'flat world' and through the process of globalization, we are now witnesses to an almost unprecedented movement of goods, services and people (including patients seeking less expensive healthcare as well as healthcare professionals and students seeking new 'experiences'), crossing national borders with much greater tendencies and frequencies than ever before.

A diverse set of subcultures (within a given culture) will then emerge from such movement of people. Such cultural developments are also likely to occur within healthcare practice between practitioners and their patients, perhaps due to patients simply misunderstanding instructions given by practitioners if a language barrier exists, or it may simply be a case of a 'clash of cultures' among practitioners themselves! Cultural tensions can then arise! In the same vein, the education environment should also expect to have students from culturally different backgrounds. How then should education respond? In Gardner's book '5 Minds for the Future',[13] he identified 'The Respectful Mind' as one of the 5 minds for the future. He said: '*The world of today and tomorrow is becoming increasingly diverse, and there is no way to cordon oneself off from this diversity. Accordingly, we must respect those who differ from us as well as those with whom we have similarities*'.

In the course of transforming students to become competent healthcare practitioners, educators must therefore instil in the minds of students the need to develop cultural sensitivity as an educational preparation for future practice. Thus, developing cultural sensitivity in students should indeed form a significant part of the curriculum of educational institutions responsible for the education of future healthcare practitioners. This will help ensure that future healthcare professionals will already be aware of the need to work with greater understanding and respect for the national characteristics of people from other lands. Such an educational preparation should lead to a more harmonious work environment in healthcare, leading to better outcomes.

Such understanding of cultural sensitivity is something that needs to be ingrained into the curriculum from Day 1. Only then can students turn habit into practice. Hence, it will be important for Ashvin and Ben to consider the sociocultural aspect of their students when planning their lessons and how this may engage with their own sociocultural identities that can influence learning outcomes. 'Importing' syllabi from other institutions often do not take into account the importance of socioeconomic-cultural context of learning within a specific setting. This can lead to suboptimal outcomes, misunderstandings and disastrous consequences due to healthcare practitioners emerging from the education system who are 'out of touch' with stakeholders across the entire spectrum of the local healthcare setting.

Selection of Specific Course Content in a Given Discipline

It is important to ensure that in the design of a curriculum, each key educational element is appropriate for the purpose intended, i.e. each key educational element must be able to collectively support the acquisition of the intended learning outcomes, which will then equip students in the medical and allied health professions courses with professional competencies that will transform them into competent healthcare practitioners upon their graduation. How then should specific course content in a given discipline be selected?

Several strategies can be used to optimise the design of a curriculum. However, the most commonly used is the Outcome Based Backward Planning and Forward Learning model.

Application of Principles Related to 'Backward Planning and Forward Learning'

'...the designer begins the process by identifying desired learning goals [outcomes for the course], and then devising [relevant strategies to deliver

instruction]... ...and assess them. Only thereafter does course-specific content come into play, and even then... ...not for the sake of 'covering' it, but as a means to achieve the previously identified learning [outcomes]. Courses designed this way put learning first... ...and usually aim to achieve more ambitious cognitive development than do classes that begin and often, end with content mastery as the primary focus. Although the advantages of backward planning are manifest, it's probably still the exception to, rather than the rule of course planning'.[14]

Today, it is vital and advantageous to apply backward planning principles in the design of a curriculum especially for undergraduate medical and health professions courses, i.e. to begin the curriculum design by, first, establishing the desired learning outcomes that students must acquire and be equipped with in order to become competent future healthcare practitioners.[15,16] The selection of specific course content and the other key educational elements will then follow and must be closely aligned to the intended learning outcomes identified for the course.

Therefore, Ashvin and Ben need to consider what are the learning goals of their lessons and whether they are aligned to the learning outcomes of the curriculum. Then, determine which content or element of their lessons will continue to deliver these goals and which will not. Curriculum in each healthcare education institution is designed to deliver the specific learning outcomes required to address the specific needs, challenges and context of a specific healthcare system. Hence, adopting the entire syllabi from other institutions designed for other healthcare contexts may, at best, not fully appreciate the local conditions and, at worst, become the antithesis to what local students really need to learn.

Optimising the Development-Design of a Curriculum For Future Medical And Healthcare Practitioners

Today, optimising the development-design of a curriculum, i.e. educational programme, for students in the medical and allied health profession courses, must be aimed at transforming students to become competent practitioners who are fit to deliver healthcare that can match the needs, demands and challenges of patients and the community.[4] Such an approach is, of course, based on the close link and the interdependence between education and practice within the healthcare delivery system.[2]

Every discipline in a professional course of study must therefore ensure that it will contribute an educational 'building block' to the overall transformative curriculum.[6] The educational 'building blocks' from various disciplines will then collectively equip the 'end-products' of education with professional competencies that will enable them to function as the new generation of competent healthcare practitioners to deliver optimal outcomes to patients and the community.

At the end of the day, it is important for the Institution'sCurriculum Committee to reach out and engage with Ashvin and Ben as well as other stakeholders such as the public and future employers for consensus planning as well as provide the necessary resources in order to design, develop and implement a curriculum that is fit for the community, embraced by the educators and engages the students. Failing which, Ashvin and Ben may feel unsupported and misunderstood. This makes them less likely to support the reformed curriculum.

Practice Highlights

- When designing, developing, organising or reforming a curriculum, the three elements to be considered are course content, instructional strategies and assessment modes.
- A curriculum must be designed to deliver the educational goals, which are in turn aligned to actual practice that is subjected to changes over time.
- A curriculum must take into consideration the socio-economic–cultural context of its learners and the environment of its graduates.
- 'Backward planning' is a potential strategy for developing a curriculum that may best serve the needs of the learners.

Key Points to Remember in the Development and Design of a Curriculum

- A curriculum is essentially an educational blueprint consisting of several key educational elements systematically organised into a learning system designed for students in a given course of study.
- A curriculum is a dynamic (not static) entity and has a 'life' of its own. It must, therefore, be updated regularly to remain relevant, i.e. adequate and appropriate to the intended course of study.
- An obsolete curriculum can cause serious 'diseases of the curriculum', e.g. 'curriculosclerosis', as well as produce ill-equipped graduates.
- The design of a curriculum must reflect the close alignment and interdependence between education and healthcare practice.
- Disruptive forces of change can impact strongly on education and practice in healthcare, and make it imperative for education and practice to undergo significant updating accordingly.

- The curriculum intended for students in the medical and allied health profession courses must be able to transform students into competent practitioners who are fit to deliver 21st-century healthcare that can meet the needs, demands and challenges of patients and the community.

References

1. Alexander L, Davis RH. Learning system design: An approach to the improvement of instruction. New York: McGraw-Hill; 1974.

2. Bligh J, Liverpool GP. Taking stock. *Medical Education.* 2000;34(6):416–7.

3. Harden RM, Sowden S, Dunn WR. Educational strategies in curriculum development: The SPICES model. *Medical Education.* 1984;18(4):284–97.

4. Frenk J, Chen L, Bhutta ZA, Cohen J, Crisp N, Evans T, et al. Health professionals for a new century: Transforming education to strengthen health systems in an interdependent world. *Lancet (London, England).* 2010;376(9756):1923–58.

5. Schuwirth LW, Van der Vleuten CP. Programmatic assessment: From assessment of learning to assessment for learning. *Medical Teacher.* 2011;33(6):478–85.

6. Miller GE. The objectives of medical education. In: Miller GE, editor. *Teaching and Learning in Medical School.* Cambridge, MA: Harvard University Press; 1961.

7. Lee TH, Duckworth AL. *Organizational grit. Harvard Business Review.* 2018.

8. Susskind R, Susskind D. *The Future of the Professions: How Technology Will Transform the Work of Human Experts.* Oxford: OUP Oxford; 2015.

9. Schwarzman SA. *Can We Make Artificial Intelligence Ethical?.* 2019 [Available from: https://www.businesstimes.com.sg/opinion/can-we-make-artificial-intelligence-ethical.

10. Samarasekera DD, Goh PS, Lee SS, Gwee MCE. The clarion call for a third wave in medical education to optimise healthcare in the twenty-first century. *Medical Teacher.* 2018;40(10):982–5.

11. Abrahamson S. Diseases of the curriculum. *Journal of Medical Education.* 1978;53(12):951–7.

12. Madara JL. Foreward. In: Hawkins RE, Lawson LE, Starr SR, Borkan J, Gonzalo JD, Skochelak SE, editors. *Health Systems Science.* 1st ed. United States: Elsevier Health Sciences; 2016.

13. Gardner H. *Five Minds for the Future.* Brighton, MA: Harvard Business School Press; 2008.

14. Burkholder P. *Backward Design, Forward Progress.* 2018 [Available from: https://www.facultyfocus.com/articles/course-design-ideas/backward-design-forward-progress/.

15. Barrow M, McKimm J, Samarasekera DD. Strategies for planning and designing medical curricula and clinical teaching. *South East Asian Journal of Medical Education.* 2010;4(1):2–8.

16. Samarasekera D, Gwee M. Building an effective training continuum in surgery: Developing a safe practitioner. *Sri Lanka Journal of Surgery.* 2013;30(2):2–10.

DELIVERY OF INSTRUCTION — 'WHY DON'T THE STUDENTS GET IT?'

Wayne Hazell, Shuh Shing Lee

Scenario

Associate Professor Chase had been a dedicated and passionate teacher for the last 20 years. He enjoyed teaching and the students also enjoyed his didactic but fun lessons. In recent years, however, he had received feedback that the students he had taught were unable to apply what they learnt to their practice. He was perplexed as to why the students could not perform in the work-based assessments since he had dutifully taught the students all that they needed to know about the subject.

Introduction

There are three interrelated elements in education: teachers, learners and contents. How well the students perform is highly dependent on what we aim to teach (the curriculum), how competent we deliver the content, equipping the students with necessary skills and arouse their curiosity to learn further (the pedagogy), and how we evaluate what students have learned (the assessment) as depicted in Fig. 1. Most of the time, knowing how to deliver the content in the curriculum poses a challenge to a teacher, especially teachers who have not trained before. Before deciding a delivery approach, understanding the learners — their characteristics and how they learn — is crucial in selecting an approach. Hence, based on the above scenario, we will first explore who our learners are? And followed by how students learn based on a few teaching and learning theories. Table 1 roughly summarises the areas that will be covered in this chapter.

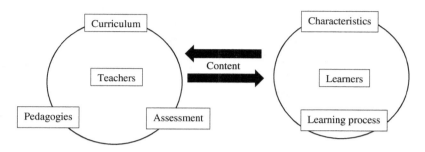

Fig. 1.   The interrelated elements in education.

Table 1.   Summary of the topics covered in this chapter.

Who our learners are?	Comparing the learning between Generations Y and Z
How do our students learn?	Based on the theories below: • Information-Processing Theory • Neurocognitive Science — Neural Plasticity • Cognitive Load Theory • Expert and Novice Learning
Factors that influence learning	Based on the theories below: • Motivation — Self-determination Theory • Affection — Pekrun's Control-value Theory

Chapter 1: Why

While we are still trying to figure out the best ways to engage Millennials, Generation Z — people who were born from 1995 onwards — they are making their presence in the higher institutions now. While both generations are considered technology-savvy generation, Generation Z uses the smartphone more frequently than a laptop as compared to millennials.[1] YouTube, Snapchat and Instagram are the top social media sites used daily among Generation Z while Facebook is most commonly used by millennials.[1] Understanding Generation Z intensely mobile-first behaviour and the social media sites that they are engaged in is the key to comprehending this generation's perception and behaviour in learning. Born with a technology device (mobile or tablet) in their hands, this interaction does change the way the brain functions and hence leading to a shorter attention span. They prefer to apply immediately what they have learned to a real-life situation after engaging in hands-on learning opportunities. The nature of technology has helped the newer generation become more comfortable and accustomed to learning independently. Whether you like it or not, being the sage on stage and delivering a lecture for hours might not be effective for students who are used to watching three-minute video clips on YouTube.[2] Therefore, educators need to acknowledge and understand that how they learn, process and retain information will be different from the previous generation.

Given that our students are more technology-savvy than the previous generation, how do the students learn? To understand this, we have to understand how our brain functions via some cognitive learning theories and neuroscience research.

Information Processing Theory

Atkinson and Shiffrin[3] advocated that the information passes our sensory organs and enters the short-term memory (STM), also known as working memory if certain attention is given. The information will be transferred to the long-term memory (LTM) if it has enough association with the existing ones or the learners have rehearsed enough to retain the information. If these processes do not occur, the information will decay from the STM (refer to Fig. 2).

Memory is conceived to be a large and permanent collection of nodes that are complexly interrelated through interacting with the environment.[4] Most of these nodes, when in LTM, are normally passive and inactive and require activation from certain 'cues' as postulated by Raaijmakers.[5] This is known as Search of Associative Memory (SAM) that describes that the storage of information is represented in memory traces or 'memory images' that contain items, associative and contextual information.[6] In order for the learners to store information and to be able to retrieve information from their LTM, the associative strengths of the new information with the existing ones have to be strong enough. In other words, if a teacher is able to help the students to connect their prior knowledge with the newly learned materials meaningfully, the information will stay in their LTM and vice versa.

The emergence of neurocognitive science has also helped us to understand learning better. The ability to learn depends on a process known as 'neural plasticity', which refers to the modification of the brain's chemistry and architecture to the environment.[7] Neurons

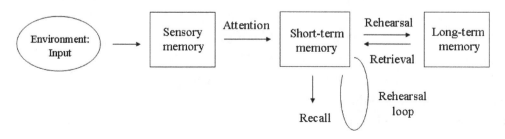

Fig. 2.   Information processing theory.

will change their structure and relationships with each other based on the experience or environment a person has gone through.[8,9] Research done by several neurocognitive science researchers on rats revealed that the cortex of the brain increases in the size, similar to the length of neurons, the number of synapses, and the level of neurotransmitters and growth hormones when they are raised in a complex and challenging environment.[10,11] Hence, the environment in nurturing or assisting students for cognitive development is essential. Some learning principles outlined by the neurocognitive scientists are not much different from the psychologists, mainly the following[7]:

- A safe and trusting relationship with an attuned other
- Maintenance of a moderate level of arousal
- Activation of both thinking and feeling
- A language of self-reflection
- Co-construction of narrative that reflects a positive and optimistic self

Cognitive Load Theory

Knowing how our information is stored and processed in LTM is insufficient to understand learning as information sometimes does not fit into the existing model especially when learners are faced with new intellectual tasks that are difficult. In order to understand how learners acquire learning, there are two critical mechanisms involved: schema acquisition and the transfer of learned procedures from controlled to automatic processing.[12]

A schema is a cognitive construct that organises the elements of information according to the manner in which they will be dealt with,[12] or in neuroscience, it is described as the effect of information on the brain that causes the neurons to form groups.[13] For example, when learners are exposed to the anatomy of structures of the limb such as ulna, radius, humeral and scapula, they are instantly incorporated into an upper limb schema instead of viewing these as an isolated entity. Hence, schema acquisition or construction of schema provides the basic unit of knowledge creation.

The second mechanism in learning is the transfer of learned procedures from controlled to automatic processing.[4,14,15] Controlled processing requires conscious attention especially involving new tasks. In contrary, automatic processing occurs without conscious control. For example, when a learner learned about lumbar puncture for the first time, the learning involved controlled processing. With time and practice, this skill will become automatic processing. Hence, as an educator, we have to understand that when a learner/student first enters the medical school or clinical years, they are dealing with huge amounts of new content or perhaps in a new environment that requires a lot of conscious attention to the materials.

Moreover, they might not be able to use previously acquired schemas to deal with a large amount of sophisticated load that has been presented to them. Based on the theory and the above scenario, is didactic lecture the best way to engage student learning?

There are three categories of cognitive load in *Cognitive Load Theory* by Sweller[16] — intrinsic, extraneous and germane. Intrinsic load is imposed by the basic structure of the information that the learners need to attend to achieve a learning goal while extraneous load refers to the manner the information is being presented to the learners. Levels by both loads are determined by the interactivity of the information (also known as an element) acquired and forming schemas in the later stage. For instance, different types of hormones in the body and their functions can be quite independently learned at different times without references to each other as this information does not interact with each other. Hence, it is considered a low level of interactivity and requires a low level of intrinsic load. Multiple small low-level schemas are built during the learning process. Unfortunately, the content/information in medicine is often highly related (such as concepts in physiology, immunology and biochemistry), which requires learners to process the information simultaneously rather than a single, unrelated matter. Such materials are not only high in interactivity but also high in intrinsic cognitive load and higher controlled processing is required.

Similarly, the extraneous cognitive load is high when unnecessary interactivity is required by a learner to process the information when it is presented in a disorganised manner (high interactivity). For example, a teacher produces a text for reading instead of providing a map/diagram in explaining how systems of human defence work might require learners to process a large amount of information simultaneously, which resulted in high interactivity and a high extraneous cognitive load. Germane load refers to the mental capacity devoted to acquire and automate schema in LTM. When we are learning something new (knowledge or skills), the experience can be daunting as we do not have the scheme to tell us what to expect and how to link to our prior knowledge. Under these circumstances, more effort and time are required to ensure the newly learned knowledge or skill forms a schema and register in LTM, resulting in a high germane load.

When the total cognitive loads (intrinsic, extraneous and germane cognitive) exceed the working memory, processing will become difficult and learning will cease. Learners will also find it exhaustive due to the highly controlled processing that takes place during the learning process and difficulty in constructing appropriate schemas. Therefore, understanding how cognitive load affects student learning enables educators to design the curriculum or content in a better fashion. Well-learned or well-organised materials can be processed automatically and reduce the cognitive load required by a learner. This will be further discussed in this chapter.

Expert and novice differences

Besides cognitive load theory, we also understand the ability to handle a different amount of information is different for individuals, especially for experts and novices. An extensive body of research has been carried out since 1980 to understand how experts learn and how do they differ from novices. Hmelo-Silver, Nagarajan, & Day,[17] in their article, summarised the differences between experts and novices from Glaser and Chi[18] research (p. 222) which are related to how information is processed as described above.

- Experts excel largely in their own domain because they have a rich base of domain knowledge.
- Experts perceive meaningful patterns in their domain of expertise reflecting a well-organised knowledge base.
- Experts are fast and accurate at solving problems within their domain because, with practice, many skills have become automated, freeing up cognitive resources for processing other aspects of the task.
- Experts represent problems at a deeper level than novices do because of their superior conceptual understanding.
- Experts spend a great deal of time analysing and representing a problem before they start solving it. This provides the experts with a cognitive representation that allow them to infer the relevant relations and constraints.
- Experts have strong self-monitoring skills.

Further evidence shows that experts store, relate and use domain knowledge differently, as opposed to novices. Experts categorise the information based on underlying principles when they are given different information, therefore, they have larger interconnected schemas. In contrast, novices view different information as similar based on surface features such as terminology. As a result, learners build multiple low-mid level schemas with limited connectivity and are unable to apply relevant concepts in learning.[19-22] When it comes to problem-solving, experts envision a problem as a whole based on the information gathered and performed an analysis based on the principles and concepts, followed by going through the details of procedures to generate a solution. Whereas novices often employ mean-end analysis in solving a problem. The learners who use this method envision the goal as a starting point and then determine the best strategy to attain the goal.[22] Therefore, when a patient is presented with a set of symptoms, novices envisage the endpoint as treating the symptoms and mapping the symptoms to different differential diagnosis as compared to experts who assemble the information and make sense of the information based on underlying principles. Experts are also more adaptable to changing context due to their highly differentiated and flexible schemas.[23] However, experts are not developed in one day and, as an educator, we cannot assume students have the same schema's structure as we do. Grooming an expert requires time and appropriate guidance along the journey.

How Motivation and Affection Affect Student Learning?

We have discussed a lot on the cognitive part of a learner especially how information is processed. However, learning also takes place while we are interacting with the environment and with peers. These interactions activate both affective and cognitive circuits that allow our brain to regulate and re-assimilate the information. In fact, emotion and motivation are some overarching concepts that influence how the learner interacts with the information provided. This will be elucidated using two relevant theories.

Many of us understand the importance of motivation in learning behaviour and that have been well-researched in general education, but not so much in medical education.[24] Within the few studies published in this area, the correlation was found between high motivation (specifically intrinsic motivation) with high academic grades in preclinical and clinical years' performance.[25,26] There are many different theories of motivation, however, we will only discuss Self-determination Theory (SDT) by Deci and Ryan[27] due to its different aspects of motivation in an individual. Deci and Ryan[27] have done extensive work in motivation and we will only provide a brief overview of the theory.

1. In order to achieve psychological growth, learners need to gain mastery of task and different skills (competence). They need to experience a sense of belonging (connection or relatedness) as well as feel in control of their own learning or behaviour (autonomy).

2. The social-contextual events (e.g. optimal challenges, effectance-promoting feedback and freedom from demeaning evaluations), which induce the feelings of competence can enhance intrinsic motivation for that action.

3. The feeling of competence will need to couple with a sense of autonomy to enhance intrinsic motivation.

4. Not only tangible rewards but also threats, directives, pressure evaluations and imposed goals diminish intrinsic motivation. In contrast, choice, acknowledgment of feelings and opportunities for self-direction were found to enhance intrinsic motivation due to greater autonomy.

5. Extrinsic motivation, as opposed to intrinsic motivation, refers to the performance of an activity to attain separable outcome which is driven by external control.

6. Motivation is a state of lacking intention to act. It can be result from not valuing an activity, not feeling competent to do it or not expecting to yield an outcome.

7. There are four types of regulation within extrinsic motivation:
   - External regulation (least autonomous) — behaviour is performed to satisfy an external demand or rewards.
   - Introjected regulation — behaviour is performed but not fully accepting it as one's own.
   - Regulation through identification — behaviour is performed with a conscious valuing of the reason behind.
   - Integrated regulation (most autonomous) — behaviour is performed after evaluation and congruence with one's other value and needs. It is fully assimilated to the self.

As learners, emotion and motivation are closely interrelated in influencing one's ability to learn. When a learner gains the desired motivation, their emotion will be positive and impart more positive energy to move forward. This is illustrated in Fig. 3.

A theory that outlines the linkages between the environment, motivation and emotion with learning in details will be Pekrun's Control Value Theory,[28] although the focus of the theory is more on emotion in learning. As depicted in Fig. 4, the environment such as support, instructional design and learners' expectation has an impact on learners' appraisal. There are two types of appraisal: the control (e.g one's ability) and value appraisals (e.g. interest) are the main determinants to the positive and negative emotions which has an effect on student motivation in learning as well as the type of learning strategies used, reciprocally emotions could also affect the appraisals. When a learner is interested in learning and expects to gain as much as they could, the outcomes that are aligned with

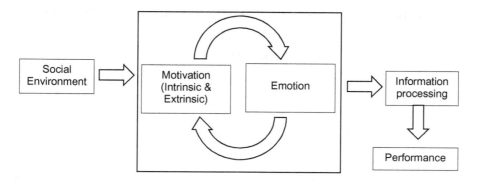

Fig. 3.   Interconnectivity of motivation and emotion in affecting one's achievement.

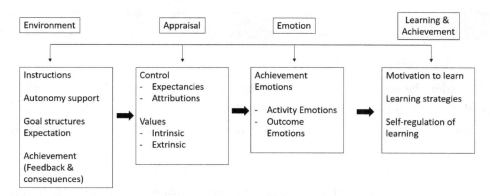

Fig. 4.   Pekrun's control value theory.

their expectation (control appraisal) and interest (value appraisal) will generate positive emotion in learning. This is known as outcome emotion. If an activity such as learning and the learning process are positively valued, enjoyment is assumed to be instigated. However, if this is negatively perceived or valued and maybe the activity is not sufficiently self-controlled, frustration is expected to arouse and learners might lose interest in learning. Therefore, all these components are actually related and you will notice some similarities with the motivational theory described above.

Understanding why the above scenario occurs and how our students learn is important to design teaching and learning activities (what to teach and how to teach). This will be the emphasis in the following chapters.

Practice Highlights

Why the above scenario occurred can be summarised in the following:

- Student learning strategies and tools to access information have evolved in the technology era.
- Teaching without understanding learners' need and learning process will be challenging for a teacher to design appropriate pedagogy that enhances meaningful learning and retention of knowledge.
- Student learning can be understood using different theories such as information-processing theory, neurocognitive science — neural plasticity, cognitive load theory, expert and novice learning.
- There are multiple factors that impact on learning, two important factors are motivation and emotion.

Chapter 2: What

Addressing the Scenario

Let's consider the scenario of Professor Chase in relation to the 'What' of delivery of instruction. There are many factors that could contribute to this outcome but what could be wrong with Professors Chase's delivery of instruction that could lead to a poor performance in his students?

This raises several important issues, but two stand out:

1. We can never assume that our teaching has the positive learning outcomes that we want until they are clearly demonstrated. This is the principle of outcome-based medical education or competency-based medical education.[29-38]

2. Medical or health professional education is a skill and/or a profession and as such education, training, continual self-reflection, peer review and evaluation are needed to acquire and maintain proficiency.[39-41]

As per Chapter 1, we will address the teacher, the student and the content.

It is assumed that these lecture sessions were face to face sessions with Professor Chase working directly with the students, although Chapter 1 has correctly identified that self-directed learning via the Internet, computers and handheld devices maybe preferred by newer generations. It appears that this feedback, assumingly from colleagues involved in assessment, has been a surprise and the reasons are unclear to him.

The teacher may or may not be a practising healthcare clinician. For the purpose of this article, we could define clinical teachers as medical or healthcare practitioners that are currently practising in their respective clinical environments while taking part in teaching students.

The students may be at a preclinical or clinical phase but ultimately the students will need learning that will set them up for clinical practice. Following on from this, the content of what is taught may be subjects forming the basis of clinical practice, such as anatomy, for example, or have direct relevance to deciding a patient's clinical plan. The student may also be postgraduate and progressing to higher or specialist qualifications.

The following content often uses clinical teachers as a focus, or comparison, for the subject matter. Please bear in mind that many principles are also applicable for any health professions educators (be it preclinical, clinical or postgraduate educators). Clinical teaching is often discussed in this chapter and Chapter 3, due to its complexities and dynamic environment. One of the authors is a medical practitioner in Emergency Medicine and experience is drawn from this setting at times.

The Teacher and Healthcare Learning Environments

Teachers deliver many, and different types of, educational sessions to healthcare students. These sessions may be in following different types of environments

- the tutorial room
- the lecture theatre
- the online environment
- the clinical environment when the teacher is working clinically at the time
- the clinical environment when the teacher is protected from clinical duties
- the simulated clinical environment

Different types of teaching delivery strategies may need to be considered in each of these environments.

Likewise, there are many different types of healthcare environments where teaching delivery can take place. Most health care clinical environments can be categorised approximately as one of the following:

1. the ward and/or the ward round
2. the operating theatre
3. outpatients, clinics or practice rooms
4. the emergency department or acute care setting
5. the community or prehospital setting
6. the home setting

Professor Chase has been giving his lectures, probably in the tutorial room or lecture theatre, but not necessarily. They may teach well in these other settings and they probably can convert or apply some of the lecture content to other settings. So, the question of *'what to deliver where arises?'* Discussion with peers interested in medical education, including a review of relevant medical education literature, can provide much idea stimulus as to what can be tried, what works and what does not work in these environments. Collections of tips from faculty can be shared and posted.

In teacher outreach programs and workshops that the authors have conducted, clinical teachers were divided into craft groups for discussion of their experience. Inevitably pearls of wisdom were offered. An example from the ward and/or the ward round group was the following:

'Before a ward round, I identify my most interesting patient for student learning.
I start the ward round with this patient and have an education session. I then
continued my round of patient care but still look out for teachable moments'[42]

As indicated in Chapter 1, the electronic, information technology, online or handheld environment is important for the newer generation learners. Full time academic or teaching staff may have the time to construct such learning but most clinical teachers may not have dedicated time to generate such resources. However, in each of the environments described above, the clinical teacher should at least have a knowledge of valuable online resources and provide motivation towards interacting with these resources. The clinical teacher can build partnerships with academic teachers that have information technology skills to create online learning platforms.[43-46]

The Teacher

After any such session in any environment, when the students leave, a teacher must ask themselves the following questions:

- *What did I do to capitalise on teachable moments?*[47]
- *What did I do well and what should I improve on?*
- *What do I need to do to improve my teaching overall?*
- *What methods did I use in relation to solid learning theory or how does my teaching relate to learning theory?*
- *What did I do to address the student's needs and questions?*
- *What did I do to make sure I was focussed on the students learning outcomes as opposed to teacher centred teaching?*[47-50]
- *How do I know my teaching style has been effective & well received?*
- *What did I do to make the teaching session memorable and did I motivate the students?*[24,51,52]
- *What did I do to check student learning or how do I know that the students have learned anything?*
- *What is the likely knowledge retention and application from my session? Have they learned what I wanted them to or have the most important items been learned?*
- *What should follow this session to maximise learning and application of learning?*
- *What have I done to align my teaching to the curriculum and assessment blueprint or strategy?*
- *What have I done to optimise my recognition of struggling students or students in difficulty?*
- *What have I done about communication with my University and course co-ordinators? Would the University and course co-ordinators be happy with how and what I am teaching? How could my University, faculty and course co-ordinators assist me with my teaching?*

If we as teachers repetitively reflect on these questions and utilise strategies or tools to close a quality assurance and educational loop, there can only be an improvement. Ultimately, the biggest what question for Professor Chase is *'What can they do to address the above-described situation?'*

In considering all of this we come to another large question: *'What makes a good teacher?'* There is also the specific question: Does Professor Chase have the characteristics associated with an effective teacher?

There is much written in the literature about the characteristics of a good teacher both in the medical and general education literature. Numerous and varied characteristics have been reported and utilised in teacher evaluation tools. An interesting question would be which of these characteristics are applicable to all forms of teaching and which are more specific to clinical teaching? Another question would be the relative importance of one characteristic in relation to others. There has been criticism of teacher characteristic sets and/or teacher evaluation tools. As this is a very complex multifactorial issue, each tool or data set may be criticised for important omissions or conversely criticised for being too detailed to be feasible.

Some evaluation tools describe characteristics that are specific to the learner's level such as medical students as opposed to residents. Although you can't help but think there must be some overlap, particularly in systems where final stage medical students are engaged in apprenticeship-style learning. Some characteristics have had importance rated by students and others have been done by teaching faculty.

Harden has put together a great summary of the teaching characteristics for effective teaching from the literature in the textbook by Harden and Liley 'The eight roles of the medical teacher. The purpose and function of a teacher in the healthcare professions'.[53] You could look at three areas of teaching: 1. Teaching abilities; 2. Approach to teaching and 3. Professionalism.[54]

Harden indicates a good teacher has some basic understanding of some educational principles, such as those outlined in Chapter 1 of this section, has evidence-informed approach and displays appropriate behaviours and attitudes. Harden and Liley,[53] list six requirements to be a good teacher:

1. Mastery of the techniques related to your work as a teacher
2. An appropriate approach to your teaching
3. Demonstration of professionalism in teaching
4. Mastery of the content of the subject to be taught
5. An understanding of the curriculum and the expected learning outcomes
6. An understanding of the different roles of a teacher

In terms of different roles of a teacher an original 12 roles has now been merged to a suggested eight[53]:

1. Information provider and coach
2. Facilitator of learning and mentor
3. Curriculum developer and implementer
4. Assessor and diagnostician
5. Role model
6. Manager and leader
7. Scholar and researcher
8. Professional

A number of collections of teacher attributes are presented in tabular form by Harden and Liley,[53] including those by Stronger,[55] Orlando[56] and Couros.[57]

The student-based identified characteristics seem to relate most to the question posed in Chapter 1 of this section: '*How motivation and affection affect student learning?*' Characteristics identified[53]:

- Passionate
- Enthusiastic about student learning
- Respects students and commit to their learning
- Empathetic, caring and compassionate
- Inspirational, motivating and encouraging
- Understanding and sensitive to learners needs
- Fair and non-judgemental
- Flexible
- Easily approachable and willing to listen
- Humorous
- Takes a personal approach and knows each student
- Humble and knows limitations

In thinking about the difference between novices and experts what are the characteristics of a teaching expert or master? This has been described by Cuoros[57] as follows:

- Connects with students and gets to know them individually
- Helps students meet their own individual needs
- Makes the curriculum and what is taught relevant
- Works with students to develop their love of learning and helps to find the students individual spark in learning
- As a teacher, keeps up to date

- Focus on learning goals as opposed to performance goals
- Ensures that character education is a part of learning. Students need to grow emotionally.
- Is passionate about the content they teach
- Concerned about not only what they teach but also about the overall impact of the school culture
- Communicates well with the stakeholders, not just the students

However, if we are thinking of clinical teachers in the clinical environment as defined above, are the characteristics similar or somewhat different? Haws's et al.[58] results suggest that the attributes of effective classroom and clinical teachers are different. Charisma and physical attractiveness are associated with the effectiveness of classroom teachers. In the clinical setting, perceived clinical skills of the teacher was the dominant attribute. This implies that the attributes of an effective teacher are context-specific and that we should not, therefore, generalise the findings from studies on teaching effectiveness from one context to another.[59] The importance of walking and talking, role modelling and having gloves on doing patient care in the clinical environment as described by Reilly[60] should not be underestimated. It may be that some clinical teachers are great in the clinical environment, some in other learning environments and some may be proficient in all environments.

In relation to considering characteristics of good teaching: What could be a common factor for preclinical teachers & clinical teachers? It may be that good preclinical teachers motivate and create direct subject relevance to future clinical practice? It may be that clinical teachers do the reverse and are able to utilise and revisit preclinical theory to assist clinical explanation?

A clinical teaching inventory rates the following factors[57]:

- Establishes a good learning environment
- Stimulates independent learning
- Allows appropriate autonomy
- Balances teaching & clinical work
- Specifies what should be learned and done
- Adjusts to learner needs
- Asks questions to promote learning
- Gives clear explanations
- Adjusts teaching to diverse settings
- Coaches in clinical and technical skills
- Incorporates research data into teaching
- Teaches clinical reasoning/diagnostic skills

- Teaches effective patient management & communication skills
- Teaches principles of cost-effective care

The evaluation and feedback for effective clinical teaching questionnaire (EFFECT) list the factors below in Table 2.[61] Many of these apply to the apprentice type model that might apply to a junior doctor but can also apply to a medical student.

There are many other tools that can be utilised for teaching evaluation or rating as evidenced by the reference list provided by Fluit and Schierkirka.[62-65] These may need to be adapted to individual settings and environments and no one tool is likely to consider all the factors that should be reflected on in a given circumstance. These tools can be biased especially if they are rated by student perception. Variance in student ratings may be explained by factors other than teaching effectiveness such as expected grades, the student's prior subject or health profession field interest, workload and difficulty, teacher or student's gender and age.[58,62-65]

Table 2. Effective clinical teaching questionnaire. (EFFECT)

Role modelling clinical skills
1. Perform history taking
2. Examine a patient
3. Perform clinical skills and procedures

Role modelling scholarship
1. Apply academic research results
2. Remodelling Can MEDS
3. Cooperate with other health professionals while providing care to patients and relatives
4. Communicate with patients
5. Cooperate with colleagues
6. Organise my own work
7. Apply guidelines and protocols
8. Treat patients respectfully
9. Handle complaints and incidents
10. Bring bad news

Role modelling professionalism
1. Indicates when he/she does not know something
2. Reflects on his/her own actions
3. Is a leading example of how I want to perform as a specialist

Table 2. (*Continued*)

Task allocation

1. Gives me enough freedom to perform tasks suiting my current knowledge/skills on my own
2. Gives me tasks that suit my current level of training
3. Stimulates me to take responsibility
4. Gives me the opportunity to discuss mistakes and incidents
5. Teaches me how to organise and plan my work
6. Prevents me from having to perform too many tasks irrelevant to my learning
7. Planning
8. Reserves time to supervise/counsel me
9. Available when I need him/her during my shift
10. Sets aside time when I need him/her
11. Quality of the feedback
12. Bases feedback on concrete observations of me
13. Indicates what I am doing correctly
14. Discusses what I can improve
15. Let me think about strengths and weaknesses
16. Reminds me of the previously given feedback
17. Formulates feedback in a way that is not condescending or insulting
18. The content of the feedback
19. My clinical and technical skills
20. How I communicate with patients
21. How I work together with my colleagues
22. How I apply for evidence-based medicine in my daily work
23. How I make ethical considerations explicit

Collegial peer review and advice with or without the aid of rating scales is another method of receiving feedback on your teaching. Some recommendations for the peer reviewer from Siddiqui et al.[41] include:

1. Choose the observer carefully
2. Set aside time for the peer observation
3. Clarify expectations
4. Familiarise yourself with the course
5. Select the instrument wisely

6. Include students
7. Be objective
8. Resist the urge to compare with your own teaching style
9. Do not intervene
10. Follow the general principles of feedback
11. Maintain confidentiality
12. Make it a learning experience

Overall a teacher, after delivering a teaching session or course, has several possible ways to consider their skills and performance:

1. Self-reflection with or without a validated rating scale. Video recordings can also be utilised to assist self-reflection
2. Student evaluation with or without a validated rating scale
3. Peer evaluation with or without a validated rating scale
4. Student assessment performance

A good teacher is also likely to use the best method approach as assisted by literature review. They will be able to pitch teaching at the right learner level whether it is a preclinical, clinical or postgraduate stage. For example, in relation to teaching the cardiovascular system in medicine at different stages you might ask **what** the best methods are to teach:

- heart sounds to a preclinical student?
- basic auscultation for cardiac murmurs in the early clinical phase?
- further ECG interpretation to late clinical phase students?
- a postgraduate specialist skill in cardiac echocardiography?

Teacher: Seek Faculty Development Opportunities

Associate Professor Chase could reflect on how he delivers his teaching through several possible faculty development options.[39,40]

If motivated, Associate Professor Chase should seek instruction in teaching delivery methods. Short teaching courses, certificates, diplomas and master's degrees are widely available. Part of the benefits from these courses is interaction with peers and discussion about teaching experiences, tips and useful resources. Many of these courses include peer review of your teaching, videoing and self-reflection on your teaching delivery.

Volunteering or applying to be an examiner or exam committee member, can provide much insight into what things should be taught e.g. looking at the steps in an OSCE assessment criteria. Conflict of interest can arise, particularly if that committee constructs examinations such as an OSCE. The teacher should seek faculty advice on how this conflict of interest is best managed with their teaching.

The Student (As Related to the Teacher)

Let's say Professor Chase gets some assistance from the faculty for development. Perhaps enrol in some teaching courses, begins to reflect on and understand the characteristics of a good teacher and their teaching practice, gets involved in peer-related discussions about best practice, and maybe even engages in peer review in different teaching settings, such that ongoing strategies are formed.

Professor Chase should now:

- eradicate long lecture sessions that are beyond the attention span of new generations
- consider other formats of teaching delivery that are likely to be more effective (see next chapter)
- understand it is not about the teacher but about the students learning (student centred teaching or learner centred teaching vs teacher centred teaching)
- recognise and effectively utilise teachable moments
- be making things memorable
- maybe incorporate some online and handheld teaching methods
- maybe even using handheld technology to get rapid learner teaching evaluation

All sounds pretty good and 'the Prof' is on the way to positive change.

However, the problem that might be still outstanding is that Professor Chase seemed to have a 'lack of awareness' that students were not meeting their learning outcomes that were linked to assessment. *'What can Professor Chase do to increase their awareness of student learning and outcomes?'*

The first step is knowing the desired outcomes that are constructively aligned to the curriculum.[66] A learning needs analysis or gap analysis of the medical students could be undertaken to have clarity around what needs to be done.[67] Strategies to heighten awareness of outcomes after a course delivery, before your colleagues recognise it before you, could include:

- Clinical direct observation and feedback prior to formal assessment. A variety of tools are available for work-based learning and assessment.
- Formative simulations, via a variety of modalities with a range of fidelities, after learning sessions (ideally with a time-gap) prior to summative assessment.
- Formative mock test situations such as a 'Mock OSCE' prior to summative assessment.
- Online self-test packages prior to summative assessment with feedback to the student and teacher.

- Being involved in formal summative assessment, either as an assistant, observer or examiner.
- Being involved in examination committees such that you can participate in the formation of examinations and then see the spread of student's performances against domains and themes.

Essentially, it is also just about knowing your students. Know something about each student by knowing their names, needs, circumstances and abilities. Know where their gaps are to assist them and how to assist them, monitor any students in difficulties, know the student who might be lacking in motivation and think of ways of motivating them, and know how your students perform in assessments.

Lastly, what we want to talk about is *'What should Professor Chase teach?'* We hear you saying that you have already advised on this; whatever is constructively aligned to the curriculum. Yes, this is nearly always true, but we will take this one step further.

Let's say you are teaching a clinical topic. It does not matter what that topic could be. It could be the assessment of a patient with abdominal pain as a doctor or back pain as a physiotherapist. The teacher can talk about a medical or health professional structure such as history or examination or drug administration, but the expert teacher often brings much more to the table, such as:

- Clinical reasoning techniques and tips
- Factors outside of the clinical script that is to play in decision-making
- Dealing with uncertainty
- Cognitive error and bias
- Communication verbal
- Communication written
- Interprofessional and interdisciplinary items
- Teamwork in general
- Teamwork in a crisis
- Reflective practice
- Professionalism in general
- Teaching about effective ways to learn
- The dialogue in relation to cognitive aids and reducing cognitive load
- Teaching about how to teach
- Motivational narratives with or without relation to personal journeys
- Links to clear significance for learners at present or in the future
- Strategies for upcoming assessments and examinations.

- Messages about self-care and wellness
- Messages about future professional pathways and responsibilities
- Cultural competency
- Generational competency

Many of the factors above are just as applicable and could be interwoven into preclinical teaching sessions as demonstrated by some clinical reasoning literature.[68]

However, could this be too difficult? As indicated above, the pitch of teaching is important to match the student stage. However, health professional students are very intelligent and highly capable individuals who can grasp concepts if they are well explained and taught. The main danger of too much or too complex concepts could be cognitive overload. The danger with too little, or not teaching the students about something that is hard, may delay learning, reduce the time they have to negotiate the learning curve, or worse still, the subject may never be considered.

Making it difficult may also have some not so obvious or counter-intuitive benefits.[69-71]

In relation to the question *'what content has Professor Chase been delivering?'* we could consider the concept of whether this has been too simple, or straightforward, even it was constructively aligned to the curriculum. Professor Chase may be delivering their lectures with a very well-structured content and a very simplified model that is well explained and easy to understand. They may be delivering it in the same environment or room every time and the students may even be comfortable and familiar with this. The students may sit back comfortably and think to themselves that this was great and the learning had come so easily and naturally to them. They may rapidly commit this to STM and they may even demonstrate their learning well if problems are posed at the time of the learning session. However, when demonstrating in the classroom, the students are drawing from their STM only. It may not indicate that they have a deep understanding of the reasoning and logic behind the learning. Real-world complexities may be ignored in order to achieve simplicity. It also does not necessarily mean that the learning will be remembered in the long term. Performance during learning does not necessarily reflect learning effectiveness.[69-71]

Desirable difficulties refer to those methods that are introduced into learning that optimise long-term learning and transfer. Having desirable difficulties introduced into students learning experiences has proven to have a considerable impact on the learner's ability to retain concepts in the long term even though such learning experiences may appear tough on the learner and at the time it may appear less effective to both the student and the teacher.

Desirable difficulties are introduced difficulties of learning such that effort and thinking are required. Working to solve a problem or expanding mental effort doing exercises that require the learners to derive principles of how to approach things in the future is likely to be far better than these principles presented to them in a simplified version upfront.[70]

Desirable difficulties may not be desired by the learners as some learners may just want a quick simplified fix or answer given by the teacher, but this is not in the learner's best interest.[70]

The 'no pain, no repetition, no gain' saying has some truth to it in learning, but it needs to be presented in a supportive way by a teacher who wants the best outcome for their health professional students. As an analogy, a teacher of army recruits should probably avoid the quick simplified lecture on how to dodge a bullet as the recruits might have to go to war one day.

If a difficult learning process leads to a well-learned framework that can be applied to many variations of the type of clinical problem presented, the learner will have the applied knowledge and skills to manage many problems and not just the one simplified by the teacher. Some difficulties experienced by learners can detract from learning. The learners must know what the method and content of desirable difficulty teaching aims to achieve, the reasons behind it and they must have the support and tools to overcome the difficulties presented.[70] Another analogy here is that you could give someone a tomato to eat for their hunger, but if you give them the skills to start and maintain a vegetable garden they will never be hungry.

As learners progress from preclinical, to clinical and postgraduate specialty the desirable difficulty concept related to reflecting real-world complexity and long-term learning transfer may be even more important. Patel et al.[72] have written about real-life contexts in relation to clinical diagnostic decision-making, and in Chapter 3, we emphasise the importance of using complex real cases to assist clinical reasoning and general decision-making.

Some content methods that may assist desirable difficulty include[70,71]:

- Varying the conditions of learning content.
- Learning content from multiple points of view.
- Interleaving content as opposed to blocking content. This is essentially mixing subject matter in a teaching session rather than blocking similar topics together. There is some evidence this leads to better long-term retention in itself, but it might seem counter-intuitive and more difficult to manage by the teacher.
- Distributing or spacing learning such that learners are pushed to recall a subject that is not at the top of their mind or tip of their tongue.
- Generation. The necessity for an idea is presented to the learner and the learners are guided to arrive at a solution.

Keeping all this in mind Professor Chase may have been well-intentioned, been trying to make things straightforward for the students by his simplified content lectures that blocked subjects nicely together. They may even have been well regarded and liked by the students for efforts to make things comfortable and the lectures rated highly by students due to this. Alas, the outcome for the students that was fed back by his colleagues!

In Chapter 3, we explore the how of teaching delivery and drill down on specific alternative methods to the 'easy' lecture and how to have a dialogue with students.

Practice Highlights

- We can never assume that our teaching has the positive learning outcomes that we want until they are clearly demonstrated.
- Medical or health professional education is a skill and/or a profession, and as such education, training, continual self-reflection, literature review, peer review, peer discussion and evaluation are needed to acquire and maintain proficiency or aim for mastery.
- There are many characteristics of effective teaching. A range of factors should be reflected on by clinical teachers in self-reflection, evaluation, peer discussion and/or peer review. This may be more useful than using individual teacher-rating scales.
- Characteristics of effective teaching may vary depending on the utilised teaching environment and it is useful to consider effective strategies in each environment.
- There are many tools that can be utilised for teaching evaluation or rating. These may need to be adapted to individual settings and no one tool is likely to consider all the factors that should be reflected on in a given circumstance. These tools can be biased especially if they are rated by student perception.
- A simple easy lecture is unlikely to contain the desirable difficulties required for long-term retention of learning.
- Consider the content range and real-life complexity of your teaching.
- Know your students.
- Explore strategies that give the teacher further information about likely student learning outcomes before the students have a summative assessment.

Chapter 3: How

How should Associate Professor Chase deliver his teaching? When considering this question, we broadly must consider a number of concepts:

- Designing and utilising learning outcomes
- Delivering on learning outcomes and checking they have been met
- Teaching modalities that could be used in these sessions
- Matching techniques to these teaching modalities
- Effective teaching delivery dialogue
- The teacher's delivery toolkit

Designing and Utilising Learning Outcomes

Many educators and learners often use the term learning objectives. There is nothing wrong with this term. However, it best describes something that is desired or needed but not necessarily guaranteed to occur as an outcome. It is best utilised when trying to understand a learner's needs and should perhaps be best avoided by teachers who are delivering sessions or courses, particularly when there are high stakes assessable outcomes that are required.

You would think Associate Professor Chase had some type of learning objectives when thinking about how their learning sessions would be constructed, but did they have clearly defined learning outcomes?

As an example of learning objectives, you are on a clinical shift and one of your health profession students can spend some time with you and your team. As a good teacher who realises that it is important to identify student needs, you to ask the medical student: 'What are your objectives for the clinical shift today?' The answers could obviously bring forth a variety of responses and the objectives raised may be: highly likely to be achievable, possibly achievable, through to very unlikely or impossible to be achieved. Learning objectives is an appropriate term in this situation. For instance, if the student says I would like to assist and participate in a lumbar puncture today the chances of this happening depends on whether the opportunity will arise with a patient scenario, whether the student is properly 'primed' for this experience, whether the clinician doing the lumbar puncture is happy to have a medical student with them, whether other learners such as junior doctors are competing for this learning experience with students and whether the patient consents for student involvement. There is no guarantee of an outcome that clinical shift, but we are not saying that this exercise is not useful. By doing this the clinical teacher now knows that they need to be on the lookout for such a clinical experience, can advise the student how to be vigilant for such a teachable moment, explore what preparation the student has for such an encounter and prepare or prime the student for such an encounter by discussion and/or by using online resources such as a lumbar puncture video.

In summary learning objectives are different from learning outcomes. They should be used in different ways. Learning objectives are best used when identifying needs when outcomes are not required or assessed, and possibly in the clinical setting due to uncontrolled variables that make outcomes uncertain. Learning outcomes are best used in planned educational sessions, courses, programs or curriculums and form the basis of outcome-based education.[29–33,66,73,74]

Similarly, they should be written in different ways. A typical learning outcome statement starts like one of the following:

1. 'At the end of the teaching session ….'
2. 'At the end of this 3-day course ….'
3. 'At the end of this 6-week speciality block or rotation ….'
4. 'At the end of the student year ….'

Professor Chase is most likely operating in one or more of the first three examples above. All these learning outcomes should then be followed by 'the health profession student will be able to'. Then this should be in turn followed by a description of the outcome desired.

In writing these learning outcomes it is useful to consider a learning level taxonomy such as Bloom's taxonomy,[75] or an adaptation or alternative to this[76,77] and consider where your outcome fits on the pyramid. Once deciding this you can select a verb that matches the desired level. See Fig. 5.

Verbs that could be utilised for each level could include[78]:

- Knowledge: defines, describes, identifies, knows, labels, lists, matches, names, outlines, recalls, recognises, reproduces, selects, states.

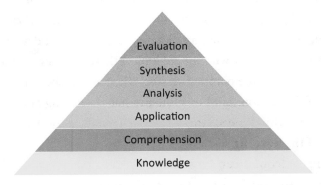

Fig. 5.   Bloom's taxonomy.[75]

- Comprehension: converts, defends, distinguishes, estimates, explains, extends, generalises, gives examples, interprets, predicts, rewrites, summarises.
- Application: applies, computes, constructs, demonstrates, discovers, operates, predicts, produces, relates, shows, solves, uses.
- Analysis: analyses, breaks down, compares, relates, selects, deconstructs, differentiates, explain, distinguishes, identifies.
- Synthesis: categorises, combines, compiles, composes, creates, devises, designs, generates, modifies, organises, plans, rearranges, reconstructs, revises, rewrites.
- Evaluation: appraise, conclude, contrast, critique.

In terms of assisting Professor Chase to think about the aspects of health professional competency, which is applicable to their learning sessions, we would direct them to the AMEE guide 14 part one and part two where a three-circle model, or Brown's nine abilities, has been described.[29,30] The aspects of the three-circle model are: 1. 'doing the right thing' or what the doctor can do; 2. 'doing the thing right' or how the doctor approaches their practice; and 3. 'the right person doing it' or professionalism. Nine abilities to consider include: 1. Effective communication; 2. Basic clinical skills; 3. Using basic science in relation to practice; 4. Diagnosis, management and prevention; 5. Lifelong learning; 6. Self-awareness, self-care and personal growth; 7. The social and community context; 8. Moral reasoning and clinical ethics; 9. Problem-solving.

If a teacher designs these learning outcomes whilst planning an educational session they can be used in several ways:

1. To make sure that the learning outcomes are constructively aligned to the curriculum. Teaching about a wide range of things is good for adult learners especially as medicine or health professions have such a broad base. However, in a planned session, compared perhaps most to a spontaneous teachable moment in an opportunistic clinical circumstance, the health profession student may not thank you for teaching something that is highly unlikely to be assessed or irrelevant to their imminent practice. Constructive alignment is about having learning outcomes that align to a declared curriculum, taught the curriculum, learned curriculum and assessed curriculum.

2. For a check by the teacher who should look at these learning outcomes upon the first draft construction of the planned session. The teacher should ask themselves given the design of the session: 'am I meeting my stated learning outcomes?' If the answer is no, one of two things needs to occur, either a rewrite of the learning outcomes or a redesign of the learning session.

3. The learning outcomes can be stated up front or given to the health profession students in the session. This way the health profession students can be orientated as

to what is to come, have clear expectations and can be thinking about meeting these outcomes through the session and further learning. The teacher can illustrate and discuss why these learning outcomes are important for future clinical practice and/ or assessment as a motivational strategy.

4. The learning outcomes can be stated again at the end of the session. Although repetitious, it is another reflective moment for both teacher and learner and another chance to emphasise the rationale for these outcomes.

5. The learning outcomes can be used in the evaluation of the session. The learners can be asked whether each outcome has been not met, partially met or met by the session.

6. The learning outcomes can be used as a reference for the teacher to decide how they can demonstrate that each student has met this outcome either in this session or subsequent sessions.

An example of how verbs linked to Bloom's taxonomy can be used in a learning session is illustrated below (Fig. 6). This learning session about curriculum construction also included learning about Bloom's taxonomy and the construction of learning outcomes. Stating the

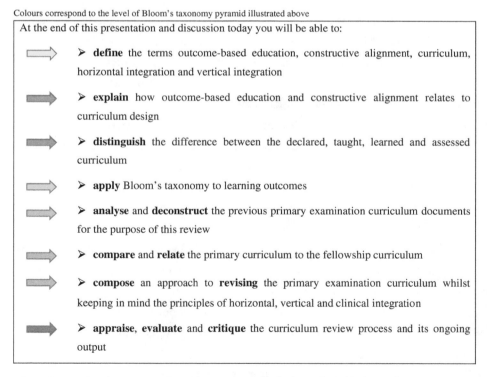

Colours correspond to the level of Bloom's taxonomy pyramid illustrated above

At the end of this presentation and discussion today you will be able to:

➢ **define** the terms outcome-based education, constructive alignment, curriculum, horizontal integration and vertical integration

➢ **explain** how outcome-based education and constructive alignment relates to curriculum design

➢ **distinguish** the difference between the declared, taught, learned and assessed curriculum

➢ **apply** Bloom's taxonomy to learning outcomes

➢ **analyse** and **deconstruct** the previous primary examination curriculum documents for the purpose of this review

➢ **compare** and **relate** the primary curriculum to the fellowship curriculum

➢ **compose** an approach to **revising** the primary examination curriculum whilst keeping in mind the principles of horizontal, vertical and clinical integration

➢ **appraise**, **evaluate** and **critique** the curriculum review process and its ongoing output

Fig. 6.   Learning session about curriculum construction, which also included learning about Bloom's taxonomy and the construction of learning outcomes.

learning outcomes whilst highlighting the verbs in a colour matched to the Bloom's taxonomy pyramid hopefully enhanced learning.[79]

Delivering on Learning Outcomes and Checking They Have Been Met

A useful exercise for those starting out in medical education is to simply request a student, or students, to demonstrate a learning outcome from a session from a week or two ago. Here is another narrative to illustrate what can happen.

Narrative 1: A training registrar in a speciality was doing a special skills term in medical education. They indicated to their medical education supervisor in the reflective discussion that the week before they had an opportunistic session in the clinical environment where they had taught a small group of students how to interpret a left bundle branch block (LBBB) on a 12-lead ECG. There was another of these sessions the following week and the medical education supervisor accompanied the trainee to provide feedback on their teaching delivery. During this second opportunistic session another patient was encountered and their ECG was relevant to the discussion. This ECG was again a LBBB and the trainee looked confidently to the supervisor and presented the ECG to the students for interpretation. However, much to the trainee's dismay, the students had much difficulty in interpreting the ECG and could not identify a LBBB.

Whilst this was very disconcerting for the up and coming clinical teacher, it provided much reflective discussion about why it could occur with the supervisor. Yes, there could be teaching delivery factors and student-related factors but are there other learning factors that we simply underestimate. As clinical teachers, particularly as experienced clinicians, we can forget how difficult it is and how much experience is required to grasp a clinical pattern or concept. It may be unreasonable to have a learning outcome, which implies fully grasping a topic or subject at the end of one learning session. Learning outcomes may need to be modified depending on the subject complexity, and the stage of the learner, to represent the stage expected on the learning curve. For the clinical teacher, we must not underestimate the value of repetition, checking for learning gaps and closing the learning gaps by further experience, practice and/or assessment. All too often we tend to give sessions on one clinical topic and move onto the next without a revisit.

The comforting messages for this novice clinical teacher were as follows:
- It is great that there was a further opportunity to check learning and close the gap further by revisiting this topic.
- There may be learning decay over time and repetition can reduce this decay. Medical students have so much to learn and all the new learning that they encounter in a

1-week period may be cognitive overload where items are competing for internal processing, understanding and recollection.[80,81]

- ECG interpretation for medical students is complex and the expectation that students may immediately grasp concepts may be unrealistic as there is much literature to suggest ECG interpretation is difficult for many levels of junior doctors up to senior registrar level.[82]

- ECG interpretation teaching is perhaps an example of desirable difficulty. Continuing the difficulty may not feel good to the teacher but it is best for long term learner outcomes.[69–71]

With this narrative, I am not suggesting that teachers now have a ready-made excuse for every learning outcome that has not been met. It is possible, and so here is another narrative to demonstrate this.

Narrative 2: A 2-week program for year four medical students (6-year course) who had a 2-week rotation in Emergency Medicine. As this was a short period, the program was designed such that they took opportunistic advantage of all learning experiences but had 10 clinical topics specifically to learn about. They would be assessed only on these 10 topics. We were confident that they could get exposure to these topics across all the four hospitals that they attended. There were clear learning outcomes, learning packages, tutorials and clinical support from clinicians familiar with teaching the ten topics. The hidden curriculum was to get the emergency medicine trainees familiar with these topics as they needed to know them for their training and would need to teach them. The students were required to have at least one real clinical encounter with a supervisor learning interaction, which would take them through the learning outcomes required. On a self-nominated repeat encounter, they then had to demonstrate their learning to show sign off of competency. In one topic, the student needed to demonstrate an adequate method of systematically reviewing a cervical spine X-ray and interpreting it correctly. Come exam time, a short answer question was submitted with a cervical spine clinical image and fracture. The overall exam coordinator felt that the question was too hard for fourth-year medical students and felt that it should be removed. The course co-ordinator felt that it had been specifically taught and learned competency had to be demonstrated by students previously. It was left in the exam post discussion and thankfully students overall did outstandingly well.[83]

The message here is that with defined learning outcomes, specific well-structured and repeated teaching targeting these learning outcomes, checking of learning and demonstration of learning, positive outcomes can be achieved. There is no doubt that narrowing the focus of the assessed curriculum was a big factor, but it was appropriate for a 2-week experience. Learning medicine and other health professions is, however, more complex than 10 topics.

So how can teachers check learning outcomes if delivering a single, or a small number of sessions, that may be a small subsection of a larger curriculum? We expand on some strategies already mentioned in Chapter 2 but these are more directly applicable to single learning sessions.

When considering these, we must reflect on desirable difficulty principles. The fact that demonstration of learning in a learning session, whilst better than no demonstration of learning and not knowing what has been learned, may not reflect long term learning and efforts to distribute or space checking learning outcomes would be optimal practice.[69-71]

These are some possible strategies to consider (in no particular order of preference or efficacy):

- Have problem-based sessions where answers to the problems can be monitored throughout and at the end of the session. The problem, which is often case based can be given to the students prior to the tutorial.
- Split sessions into two halves: one learning and one demonstration of learning.
- Follow small group tutorials with simulations on the same subject.
- Follow small group session with directly observed learning such as a Mini-CEX or DOPS.
- Like the above, if you have sequential sessions, have a small group tutorial one week and a demonstration of learning the following week perhaps by doing another problem-based case that targets similar learning outcomes.
- Split sessions into three parts:
  1. A simulated clinical experience prior to any tutorial to identify what is known, what is not known and the learning needs. This can be a motivation for the students to learn in the following two parts.
  2. A small group tutorial, which addresses this and planned learning outcomes.
  3. Repeat a simulated experience to check learning.
- End sessions with a brief MCQ or short answer assessment. Online or handheld apps could be utilised here.
- Get students to write down what they have learned, what they have had difficulty with and what questions they have at the end of a session. This can be anonymous, submitted and followed up at a subsequent session.
- Advise students that at the next session they will be asked about certain things to check their learning and/or at a subsequent session get students to write down or put on a whiteboard what they have learned from the previous week.

To reinforce what has been learned from experience in the clinical environment and relate this to course curriculum, learning outcomes can be checked by:

- Case presentations: Referring to the curriculum visually during this can be helpful.
- Learning and experiential portfolios that are reviewed by clinical teachers.
- Workplace-based assessment and learning events (WBA, WBL, WBAL).

Throughout a more prolonged period, or a course, there is more opportunity perhaps to check and provide feedback on learning outcomes at designated spots on the way through which is a type of programmatic assessment.[84]

Teaching Modalities That Could Be Used in These Sessions

In the scenario, it is noted that Associate Professor Chase has been utilising didactic teaching sessions. The age-old myth that we retain 10% of what we read, 20% of what we hear, 30% of what we see, 50% of what we see and hear, 70% of what is discussed with others, 80% of what we experience and 95% of what we teach has largely been debunked for many reasons including that such research to get such precise figures would just not be possible.[85] However, the concept of active participation in learning activities related to prescribed learning outcomes being more effective than a student passively listening to a lecturer is well founded and described in chapters by Biggs.[66]

Didactic teaching is also a mostly teacher centred method of teaching delivery. The method here is that the teacher is more mindful of showing their prowess in their grasp of the clinical subject and putting on a 'how good am I' performance such that the learners' needs, and questions, are not as important. The teacher may seek to demonstrate their knowledge but not think about how best to break it down and explain it to the students. The teacher is likely to deliver the education to suit their own learning style but not consider the differing learning styles of their students nor the best ways to help them process the information.[66]

Small group session that includes active participation, discussion, reflection, problem-solving and doing have been shown to be more closely related to improved learning outcomes.

Reasons to use small group education according to Walton[86] may include:

- Difficult subject matter and complex clinical concepts can be grasped more easily if learners can raise their own questions and needs (deep as opposed to superficial learning [66])
- Knowledge, problem-solving and decision-making can be subjected to reasoning
- Attitudes and biases may become evident
- Interaction with peers and colleagues may increase motivation

- The opportunity to learn from each other can allow a learner to keep pace with rapid changes in all branches of medicine and have a deeper grasp of the subject matter
- Counteracts any authority gradient between the teacher and learner
- Allows reflection on and examination of the learner's behaviour
- Fosters the ability to work in a team, which is now an absolute requirement for a health professional
- They can witness the effect they have on other individuals and have feedback on this. Groups can also modify an individual's behaviour.
- Improve one's problem-solving skills, critical thinking, reflection and reasoning

The effectiveness of the session is dependent on the discussion skills of the tutor and students. Asking questions, listening, responding, explaining, opening and closing, and preparation done well can lead to improved cognitive skills of students such as gaining understanding, critical thinking, reasoning, problem-solving, decision-making and creative thinking.[86-88]

There are many types of small group sessions. There the only end to the different uses, types, and formation is the limitation of the teacher's imagination as applied to the purpose of the education. Small group teaching can be structured around topics or themes, clinical cases, clinical problems (Problem-Based Learning: PBL), journal articles, situations, tasks and skills. There can be many formats such as games, controlled discussion, step by step, associative discussion, team-based learning, workshops, seminars, milling, rounds, buzz groups, three minutes each way, snowball groups, fishbowl groups, role play, five-minute theatre, paired feedback, representatives observed, hot seat for the tutor, crossover group, circular question and post-event or simulation debriefing, syndicates or project groups, electronic groups such as videoconferencing or blogging.[86-90]

Tips for effective small group teaching from Steinert[91] include:

1. Plan ahead:
   - consider the many uses of small groups
   - formulate clear objectives and a possible 'map' for the teaching session
   - determine group size and arrange the physical facilities
2. Convene the group and develop a mutually acceptable agenda:
   - introduce group members to each other
   - assess student needs and expectations
   - develop a group agenda
3. Create a positive atmosphere for learning
4. Focus the group on the task at hand

5. Promote individual involvement and active participation:
   - question effectively listen attentively
   - reinforce student contributions
6. Vary the teaching methods
7. Provide relevant information and respond appropriately
8. Observe and clarify group process
9. Work to overcome commonly encountered problems
10. Synthesise and summarise the group discussion
11. Evaluate the session and plan for follow up
12. Enjoy yourself and have fun!

The AMEE Guide No. 48. Effective small group learning,[92] has a list of common errors or problems that need to be prevented or overcome in small group teaching. These include:
- 'Tutors talk too much'
- Low level of participation
- Tutor-centred class when it should be student-centred
- Discussion dominated by a few students
- Low level of discussion
- Too many questions
- Questions rarely rise above the level of recall
- The discussion is unintentionally unfocused
- Insufficient variety of activities in a session
- Poor preparation by students
- Not sufficient or poor feedback to students
- Insufficient or inappropriate use of equipment
- Inability or unwillingness of tutors to respond to questions
- Little attempt to get students to answer their own questions

Effective Delivery Dialogue

In relation to small group tutorials, the AMEE guide 48 makes the practice points that 'questioning, listening and responding are key skills for tutors and students to develop'. 'Facilitating methods' and 'attention to the dynamic of the group is important'. It is essentially about the dialogue of the teacher facilitating dialogue from the students leading to gaining understanding, critical thinking, reasoning, problem-solving, decision-making and creative thinking.[92]

This concept has much wider applicability than just small group tutorials and can be used in any setting where there is dialogue with a student including the clinical settings and debriefing after simulated clinical encounters.

Let's consider some questions and techniques that a clinical teacher can use. A student asks you a question. How should you respond? A good first up rule is to try not to answer a question with an immediate answer. If you immediately answer you might have prevented the student thinking through the problem themselves, or not understand why they are asking that question, or prevent them making a commitment to a clinical decision such that they will learn whether their clinical judgment is right or wrong. You may also not engage other students in the discussion. The best thing to do is often pose a question to a question. Some possible replies to this could be:

- What do you think could be the answer?
- What do you think should be done in that circumstance?
- Can the group help us out discussing the answer to that question?
- What is the background to you asking that question?

These questions ultimately lead to more discussion and thinking, and the clinical teacher can gain insight into the where the students are at in relation to the topic, as well as listening carefully to their thought processes to gauge whether they have sound reasoning skills. Various information will come out in that discussion and depending on where things end, the teacher may just need to reaffirm correct thoughts or correct minor misconceptions. Sometimes, of course, the teacher may need to inform knowledge gaps or give references or strategies to do so.

This needs to be done in a safe environment with some ground rules where the students don't feel threatened by participating in the discussion and possibly being wrong. A good dialogue from the teacher can be something like:

- 'Don't be afraid to be wrong'
- 'It is OK to be wrong here'
- 'It is OK to be wrong, but it is not OK to not have a go'

It is important to a student or groups of students to commit to an answer to a problem. In the clinical setting, when a student is presenting a case, this can be done via the five step micro-skills process. The 5 steps here being[93]:

1. Get a commitment
2. Probe for supporting evidence
3. Teach general rules
4. Reinforce what was done right
5. Correct mistakes

In the small group setting, there is some potential dialogue that can be helpful regarding commitment. As examples:

- 'Committing to an answer helps you learn about your clinical judgment and applied knowledge'.
- 'After a clear commitment which requires active thinking, feedback and reflection on whether you are wrong, or right is a powerful and memorable learning experience'.

In small group sessions, there are some techniques that can assist commitment and relate this to clinical reasoning. Take for instance an evolving real case presentation where students are trying to hone their diagnostic reasoning skills. At a point in the tutorial, the clinical teacher could ask the students, in turn, to commit to their most likely diagnosis. After a range of diagnoses, the teacher could go back to each student and ask them what supports their most likely diagnosis and is there any factors that weigh against it. The case plays out and the students learn the diagnosis with further discussion around the weighed factors and process leading to this conclusion.

Exploratory and probing dialogue by the teacher is recommended. A range of why; how and what questions could be utilised. Why have you put that diagnosis on top of your differential? What are the underlying principles? How reliable is the evidence supporting that practice?[92]

When using dialogue to explore problem-solving and clinical reasoning it is useful to consider some models and related questioning dialogue.

When trying to solve a problem there are eight elemental structures of thought[94]:

1. We think for a PURPOSE
2. Within a POINT OF VIEW
3. Based on ASSUMPTIONS
4. With IMPLICATIONS & CONSEQUENCES
5. We use DATA, FACTS & EXPERIENCE
6. To make INFERENCES or JUDGEMENTS
7. Based on CONCEPTS & THEORIES
8. To answer a QUESTION

An example of exploratory questions matched to each of the eight items above could be:

1. What is the objective of your clinical reasoning?
2. What is your unique point of view and what other points of view should be considered in reasoning through this problem?
3. Have you made any assumptions in this reasoning? Is it safe to use that assumption?

4. Given your assumptions what are the implications and consequences if those assumptions are wrong?

5. What additional data do we need to make a safe decision? Can we turn an assumption into a fact by getting more data?

6. Are there any grey areas where you have had to use your clinical judgment in your decision-making? If so, explain your reasoning behind this judgment.

7. What key concepts and theories are guiding your clinical reasoning?

8. What is the most important clinical question to answer?

Similarly, when trying to analyse whether a student's argument is logical we need to think about nine factors consistent with the 'Universal Intellectual Standards' of sound clinical reasoning, which are[94]:

1. Clarity
2. Accuracy
3. Precision
4. Relevance
5. Depth
6. Breadth
7. Logic
8. Significance
9. Fairness

The clinical teacher can use questioning and dialogue around these aspects to guide the student toward logical thinking. As examples[94]:

1. Clarity: I am not completely clear what you mean here. Can you explain and illustrate this in more detail so I can understand?

2. Accuracy: How could we verify whether that is correct information?

3. Precision: Could you give me more specific details surrounding that?

4. Relevance: How does that relate to the patients presenting problem?

5. Depth: What are some of the complex decisions we need to make in the setting of this condition?

6. Breadth: Do we need to consider any other conditions, or could we need to look at this in other ways?

7. Logic: Does this make sense when we weigh up all the information?

8. Significance: What is the highest priority with this patient's management? Or what piece of history has the highest significance in making our conclusion?

9. Fairness: Am I being sympathetic to the viewpoint of the patient?

Talking or thinking aloud is a useful method for the clinical teacher to utilise in dialogue. This method involves the expert or the clinical teacher breaking down their rationale step by step when problem-solving and saying this aloud to the students. It is essentially an insight into the inner workings of an expert's mind. Similarly, the clinical teacher should use dialogue to encourage the student thinking aloud such that the teacher can fully understand this thinking and give educational feedback.[95]

We would usually recommend the use of real cases in clinical reasoning. The following is a checklist, over and above the eight elemental structures of thought and the Universal Intellectual Standards, to consider when constructing case narratives for thinking aloud or clinical reasoning teaching (see Table 3).

The other very powerful aspect of teaching is feedback.[96] In the group setting, where other students will hear feedback, it is extremely important to give feedback in such a way that it is not personal. The best way to do this is giving feedback directly related to the problem being discussed. If there is sensitive or behavioural feedback to be given it may be best done after the session on an individual basis. Feedback should follow the following principles[97]:

- An informed, non-evaluative, objective appraisal
- Aimed at improving clinical skills or performance rather than estimating personal worth
- Clarifies what is good performance
- Provides opportunities to close the gap between current and desired performance
- Specific in that reasons why are given in relation to what has been observed

Table 3.   Suggested checklist for components of real cases used for think aloud and clinical reasoning teaching.

- Deductive vs Heuristic reasoning
- Progressive responsibility in decision-making
- Systems, situations, and settings in relation to clinical decision-making.
- Identification of what decisions need to be made
- Identification of time frames required for these decisions
- Dealing with uncertainty
- Identification of priorities
- Recognising error-prone situations
- Avoidance strategies to prevent error
- Principles of Evidence-Based Medicine
- Professionalism

- Immediate and formative
- Facilitates the development of self-assessment, and reflection in learning
- Encourages positive motivational beliefs and esteem; positive feedback and reinforcement should not be forgotten

Finally, Table 4 outlines some potential working rules for teaching dialogue:

Table 4. Teaching dialogue delivery.

1. Create a safe environment where it is OK to be wrong.
2. Try not to answer a question with an immediate answer. Pose a question to a question to further facilitate discussion.
3. Involve the student group in answering questions posed by a student.
4. Get a commitment from the students before discussion and answers.
5. Use exploratory and probing dialogue to facilitate further discussion and explore clinical reasoning.
6. Talk or think aloud such that the students can clearly see your clinical reasoning.
7. Facilitate the students talking or thinking aloud such that you can clearly see their clinical reasoning.
8. Utilise the principles of effective feedback.

Practice Highlights

How a teacher should address the above scenario with their teaching delivery could include the following:

- Construct and utilise learning outcomes in planned education sessions.
- Ensure planned teaching sessions are constructively aligned to the declared and assessed curriculum.
- Utilise small group teaching methods that involve active discussion & problem-solving; reflection on real or simulated clinical experiences; direct observation of students applying knowledge, skills and professional attributes; assessments designed for learning prior to any formal assessment; and incorporation of principles of desirable difficulty.
- Have a toolkit of strategies when having a dialogue with students to encourage reflection and active thinking.

- Consider working rules and clinical reasoning frameworks and narratives, that can be widely applied across planned educational sessions and teachable moments
- Devise a range of strategies to check on learners needs, gaps and what has been learned

References

1. Kleinschmit M. *Generation Z Characteristics: 5 Infographics on the Gen Z Lifestyle*; 2019.

2. Jermyn D. How colleges are adapting for the new Gen Z. *The Globe and Mail*. 2018.

3. Atkinson RC, Shiffrin RM. Human memory: A proposed system and its control processes. *Psychology of Learning and Motivation*. 1968;2:89–195.

4. Shiffrin RM, Schneider W. Controlled and automatic human information processing: II. Perceptual learning, automatic attending, and a general theory. *Psychological Review*. 1977;84(2):127–90.

5. Raaijmakers JG. *Retrieval from Long-term Store: A General Theory and Mathematical Models: [Sl: sn]*; 1979.

6. Raaijmakers JGW. Spacing and repetition effects in human memory: Application of the SAM model. *Cognitive Science*. 2003;27(3):431–52.

7. Cozolino L, Sprokay S. Neuroscience and adult learning. *New Directions for Adult and Continuing Education*. 2006;2006(110):11–19.

8. Buonomano DV, Merzenich MM. Cortical plasticity: From synapses to maps. *Annual Review of Neuroscience*. 1998;21:149–86.

9. Trojan S, Pokorný J. Theoretical aspects of neuroplasticity. *Physiological Research*. 1999;48(2):87–98.

10. Guzowski JF, Setlow B, Wagner EK, McGaugh JL. Experience-dependent gene expression in the rat hippocampus after spatial learning: A comparison of the immediate-early genes Arc, c-fos, and zif268. *The Journal of Neuroscience*. 2001;21(14):5089–98.

11. Ickes BR, Pham TM, Sanders LA, Albeck DS, Mohammed AH, Granholm AC. Long-term environmental enrichment leads to regional increases in neurotrophin levels in rat brain. *Experimental Neurology*. 2000;164(1):45–52.

12. Sweller J. Cognitive load theory, learning difficulty, and instructional design. *Learning and Instruction*. 1994;4(4):295–312.

13. Legendy CR. On the scheme by which the human brain stores information. *Mathematical Biosciences*. 1967;1(4):555–97.

14. Schneider W, Shiffrin RM. Controlled and automatic human information processing: I. Detection, search, and attention. *Psychological Review*. 1977;84(1):1.

15. Kotovsky K, Hayes JR, Simon HA. Why are some problems hard? Evidence from Tower of Hanoi. *Cognitive Psychology*. 1985;17:248–94.

16. Sweller J. *Cognitive Load Theory*. Academic Press; 2011:37–76.

17. Hmelo-Silver CE, Nagarajan A, Day RS. "It's harder than we thought it would be": A comparative case study of expert-novice experimentation strategies. *Science Education*. 2002;86(2):219–43.

18. Glaser R, Chi MTH. Overview. In: Chi MTH, Glaser R, Farr MJ, editors. *The Nature of Expertise.* Hillsdale, NJ: Lawrence Erlbaum Associates, Inc; 1988:xxxvi, 434-xxxvi.

19. Chi MTH, Feltovich PJ, Glaser R. Categorization and representation of physics problems by experts and novices. *Cognitive Science.* 1981;5:121–152.

20. Hardiman PT, Dufresne R, Mestre JP. The relation between problem categorization and problem solving among experts and novices. *Memory & Cognition.* 1989;17(5):627–38.

21. Schoenfeld AH, Herrmann DJ. Problem perception and knowledge structure in expert and novice mathematical problem solvers. *Journal of Experimental Psychology: Learning Memory and Cognition.* 1982;8(5):484–94.

22. Dufresne R, Gerace W, Hardiman P, Mestre J. Constraining novices to perform expertlike problem analyses: Effects on schema acquisition. *The Journal of the Learning Sciences.* 1992;2(3):307–31.

23. Feltovich PJ, Spiro RJ, Coulsen RL. Issues of expert flexibility in contexts characterized by complexity and change. In: Feltovich PJ, Ford KM, Hoffman RR, editors. *Expertise in Context.* Menlo Park, CA: AAAI Press; 1997:125–46.

24. Kusurkar RA, Ten Cate TJ, van Asperen M, Croiset G. Motivation as an independent and a dependent variable in medical education: A review of the literature. *Medical Teacher.* 2011;33(5):e242–62.

25. Sobral DT. What kind of motivation drives medical students' learning quests? *Medical Education.* 2004;38(9):950–7.

26. Moulaert V, Verwijnen MGM, Rikers R, Scherpbier AJJA. The effects of deliberate practice in undergraduate medical education. *Medical Education.* 2004;38(10):1044–52.

27. Deci EL, Ryan RM. *Intrinsic Motivation and Self-determination in Human Behavior.* New York: Plenum; 1985.

28. Pekrun R, Frenzel AC, Goetz T, Perry RP. The control-value theory of achievement emotions: An integrative approach to emotions in education. In: Schutz PA, Pekrun R, editors. *Emotion in Education.* Elsevier; 2007:13–36.

29. Harden RM, Crosby JR, Davis MH. Amee guide no. 14: Outcome-based education: Part 1-an introduction to outcome-based education. *Medical Teacher.* 1999;21(1):7–14.

30. Smith SR. AMEE Guide No. 14: Outcome-based education: Part 2-Planning, implementing and evaluating a competency-based curriculum. *Medical Teacher.* 1999;21(1):15–22.

31. Ben-David M. Amee guide no. 14. Outcome-based education: Part 3-assessment in outcome-based education. *Medical Teacher.* 1999;21(1):23–5.

32. Ross N, Davies D. Amee guide no. 14. Outcome-based education: Part 4-outcome-based learning and the electronic curriculum at Birmingham medical school. *Medical Teacher.* 1999;21(1):26–31.

33. Harden RM, Crosby JR, Davis MH, Friedman M. Amee guide no. 14: Outcome-based education: Part 5-from competency to meta-competency: A model for the specification of learning outcomes. *Medical Teacher.* 1999;21(6):546–52.

34. Rosenberg ME. An outcomes-based approach across the medical education continuum. *Transactions of the American Clinical and Climatological Association.* 2018;129:325.

35. Holmboe ES, Batalden P. Achieving the desired transformation: Thoughts on next steps for outcomes-based medical education. *Academic Medicine.* 2015;90(9):1215–23.

36. Gruppen LD. Outcome-based medical education: Implications, opportunities, and challenges. *Korean Journal of Medical Education.* 2012;24(4):281–5.

37. Holmboe ES. Competency-based medical education and the ghost of Kuhn: Reflections on the messy and meaningful work of transformation. *Academic Medicine.* 2018;93(3):350–3.

38. Caverzagie KJ, Nousiainen MT, Ferguson PC, ten Cate O, Ross S, Harris KA, et al. Overarching challenges to the implementation of competency-based medical education. *Medical Teacher.* 2017;39(6):588–93.

39. Leslie K, Baker L, Egan-Lee E, Esdaile M, Reeves S. Advancing faculty development in medical education: A systematic review. *Academic Medicine.* 2013;88(7):1038–45.

40. Dath D, Iobst W, Collaborators IC. The importance of faculty development in the transition to competency-based medical education. *Medical Teacher.* 2010;32(8):683–6.

41. Siddiqui ZS, Jonas-Dwyer D, Carr SE. Twelve tips for peer observation of teaching. *Medical Teacher.* 2007;29(4):297–300.

42. Henning M, Hazell W. An interactive and reflective series of sessions aimed to enhance effective clinical teaching. 9th Asia Pacific Medical Education Conference 11 January 2012; National University of Singapore; 2011.

43. Lim EC, Oh VM, Koh DR, Seet RC. Harnessing the IT factor in medical education. *Annals Academy of Medicine Singapore.* 2008;37(12):1051.

44. Kho A, Henderson LE, Dressler DD, Kripalani S. Use of handheld computers in medical education. *Journal of General Internal Medicine.* 2006;21(5):531–7.

45. Masters K, Ellaway RH, Topps D, Archibald D, Hogue RJ. Mobile technologies in medical education: AMEE Guide No. 105. *Medical Teacher.* 2016;38(6):537–49.

46. Duncan I, Yarwood-Ross L, Haigh C. YouTube as a source of clinical skills education. *Nurse Education Today.* 2013;33(12):1576–80.

47. Chinai SA, Guth T, Lovell E, Epter M. Taking advantage of the teachable moment: A review of learner-centered clinical teaching models. *Western Journal of Emergency Medicine.* 2018;19(1):28.

48. Ebert-May D, Derting TL, Henkel TP, Middlemis Maher J, Momsen JL, Arnold B, et al. Breaking the cycle: Future faculty begin teaching with learner-centered strategies after professional development. *CBE—Life Sciences Education.* 2015;14(2):ar22.

49. Savoy M, Yunyongying P. Can a simplified approach to emotional intelligence be the key to learner-centered teaching? *Journal of Graduate Medical Education.* 2014;6(2):211–4.

50. Menachery EP, Wright SM, Howell EE, Knight AM. Physician-teacher characteristics associated with learner-centered teaching skills. *Medical Teacher.* 2008;30(5):e137–e44.

51. Regan-Smith M, Hirschmann K, Iobst W. Direct observation of faculty with feedback: An effective means of improving patient-centered and learner-centered teaching skills. *Teaching and Learning in Medicine.* 2007;19(3):278–86.

52. Ramani S. Memorable outpatient teaching: The sum of many teachable moments. *Medical Teacher.* 2015;37(10):971–3.

53. Harden RM, Lilley P. *The Eight Roles of the Medical Teacher — The Purpose and Function of a Teacher in the Healthcare Professions*. United Kingdom: Elsevier; 2018.

54. Harden RM, Laidlaw JM. *Essential Skills for a Medical Teacher: An Introduction to Teaching and Learning in Medicine*. United Kingdom: Elsevier Health Sciences; 2016.

55. Stronge JH. *Qualities of Effective Teachers: Association for Supervision and Curriculum Development*; 2007.

56. Orlando M. *Nine Characteristics of a Great Teacher*. Faculty Focus.

57. Cuoros G. *What Makes a Master Teacher? The Principles of Change*; 2010.

58. Haws J, Rannelli L, Schaefer JP, Zarnke K, Coderre S, Ravani P, et al. The attributes of an effective teacher differ between the classroom and the clinical setting. *Advances in Health Sciences Education: Theory and Practice*. 2016;21(4):833–40.

59. van der Vleuten CP. When I say... context specificity. *Medical Education*. 2014;48(3):234–5.

60. Reilly BM. Inconvenient truths about effective clinical teaching. *Lancet (London, England)*. 2007;370(9588):705–11.

61. Copeland HL, Hewson MG. Developing and testing an instrument to measure the effectiveness of clinical teaching in an academic medical center. *Academic Medicine*. 2000;75(2):161–6.

62. Fluit C, Bolhuis S, Grol R, Ham M, Feskens R, Laan R, et al. Evaluation and feedback for effective clinical teaching in postgraduate medical education: Validation of an assessment instrument incorporating the CanMEDS roles. *Medical Teacher*. 2012;34(11):893–901.

63. Fluit CR, Feskens R, Bolhuis S, Grol R, Wensing M, Laan R. Understanding resident ratings of teaching in the workplace: A multi-centre study. *Advances in Health Sciences Education*. 2015;20(3):691–707.

64. Schiekirka S, Feufel MA, Herrmann-Lingen C, Raupach T. Evaluation in medical education: A topical review of target parameters, data collection tools and confounding factors. *German Medical Science: GMS e-journal*. 2015;13:Doc15.

65. Schiekirka S, Raupach T. A systematic review of factors influencing student ratings in undergraduate medical education course evaluations. *BMC Medical Education*. 2015;15(1):30.

66. Biggs J, Tang C. *Teaching for Quality Learning at University: What the Student Does*. 4th ed. New York: Society for Research into Higher Education and Open University Press; 2011.

67. Hazell W. Where to now after a learning and educational needs analysis of Fellows of the Australasian College for Emergency Medicine? *Emergency Medicine Australasia*. 2008;20(2):101–4.

68. Min Simpkins AA, Koch B, Spear-Ellinwood K, St John P. A developmental assessment of clinical reasoning in preclinical medical education. *Medical Education Online*. 2019;24(1):1591257.

69. Weissgerber SC, Reinhard M, Schindler S. Learning the hard way: Need for cognition influences attitudes toward and self-reported use of desirable difficulties. *Educational Psychology*. 2018;38(2):176–202.

70. Anand P. Difficulties in learning. *Training Journal*. 2015;3:31–3.

71. Gaspelin N, Ruthruff E, Pashler H. Divided attention: An undesirable difficulty in memory retention. *Memory & Cognition*. 2013;41(7):978–88.

72. Patel R, Sandars J, Carr S. Clinical diagnostic decision-making in real life contexts: A trans-theoretical approach for teaching: AMEE Guide No. 95. *Medical Teacher*. 2015; 37(3):211–27.

73. Houlden RL, Collier CP. Learning outcome objectives: A critical tool in learner-centered education. *Journal of Continuing Education in the Health Professions*. 1999;19(4):208–13.

74. Morcke AM, Dornan T, Eika B. Outcome (competency) based education: An exploration of its origins, theoretical basis, and empirical evidence. *Advances in Health Sciences Education*. 2013;18(4):851–63.

75. Bloom BS. *Taxonomy of Educational Objectives, Vol. 1: Cognitive Domain*. New York: McKay. 1956:20–4.

76. Muehleck JK, Smith CL, Allen JM. Understanding the advising learning process using learning taxonomies. *NACADA Journal*. 2014;34(2):63–74.

77. Irvine J. A comparison of revised bloom and marzano's new taxonomy of learning. *Research in Higher Education Journal*. 2017;33:1–16.

78. Stanny CJ. Reevaluating bloom's taxonomy: What measurable verbs can and cannot say about student learning. *Education Sciences*. 2016;6:1–12.

79. Hazell WC. Primary exam curriculum review workshop. [Personal communication from slide programme and from education session]. In press 2009.

80. Yang J, Zhan L, Wang Y, Du X, Zhou W, Ning X, et al. Effects of learning experience on forgetting rates of item and associative memories. *Learning & Memory*. 2016;23(7):365–78.

81. Pertzov Y, Manohar S, Husain M. Rapid forgetting results from competition over time between items in visual working memory. *Journal of Experimental Psychology: Learning, Memory, and Cognition*. 2017;43(4):528–36.

82. Hazell W. Level of practice for ECG interpretation skills should be 'expert'. *Emergency Medicine Australasia*. 2007;19(2):81–5.

83. Hazell WC. The Yr 4 Undergraduate Emergency Medicine Logbook Project. [Personal communication in relation to course assignment]. In press 2010.

84. Schuwirth LWT, Van der Vleuten CPM. Programmatic assessment: From assessment of learning to assessment for learning. *Medical Teacher*. 2011;33(6):478–85.

85. *Learning Retention Rates*. Brisbane, Australia: The Peak Performance Centre; 2019.

86. Walton H. Small group methods in medical teaching. *Medical Education*. 1997;31(6):459–64.

87. Ahmed MU, Roy S. Small group teaching-an update. *Bangladesh Journal of Medical Microbiology*. 2014;8(8):28–31.

88. *UCD Teaching and Learning Downloadable Resources Toolkit: Large and Small Group Teaching*. University College Dublin; 2019.

89. Ferris H. The use of small group tutorials as an educational strategy in medical education. *International Journal of Higher Education*. 2015;4:226–8.

90. Meo SA. Basic steps in establishing effective small group teaching sessions in medical schools. *Pakistan Journal of Medical Sciences*. 2013;29(4):1071–6.

91. Steinert Y. Twelve tips for effective small-group teaching in the health professions. *Medical Teacher.* 1996;18(3):203–7.

92. Edmunds S, Brown G. Effective small group learning: AMEE Guide No. 48. *Medical Teacher.* 2010;32(9):715–26.

93. Neber JO, Gordon KC, Meyer B, Stevens N. A five-step "microskills" model of clinical teaching. *Journal of the American Board of Family Practice.* 1992;5:419–24.

94. Hawkins DR, Paul R, Elder L. *The Thinker's Guide to Clinical Reasoning: Foundation for Critical Thinking.* The Foundation for Critical Thinking; 1st edition; 2010.

95. Pinnock R, Young L, Spence F, Henning M, Hazell W. Can think aloud be used to teach and assess clinical reasoning in graduate medical education? *Journal of Graduate Medical Education.* 2015;7(3):334–7.

96. Hattie J, Timperley H. The Power of Feedback. *Review of Educational Research.* 2007;77(1):81–112.

97. *Principles of Effective Feedback.* London Deanery; 2019.

ASSESSMENT: 'HOW CAN I ASSESS FOR MY TRAINEE TO PERFORM BETTER?'

Gominda G Ponnamperuma, Lambert W.T. Schuwirth

Scenario

The graduates of *Excellence for Life* School of Medicine were awarded a degree, which certified that they possessed the necessary professional competence. However, when they started their practice, the healthcare team members complained that the graduates had major gaps in communication and some core procedural skills. The graduates countered that they had passed all tests related to these communication and procedural skills and had a degree that guaranteed that they had the requisite competences.

Introduction

'The unexamined life is not worth living' (Socrates).

'The unexamined exam is not worth interpreting' (with apologies to Socrates).

An examination of an exam involves exploring the 'why', 'what' and 'how' pertaining to that exam. Before exploring these, however, an examination of the philosophical basis of assessment will be helpful to clarify some of the core theoretical underpinnings of assessment. Hence, the following explanation of the underlying rationale of assessment will serve as an essential introduction to the three chapters of assessment that follow.

If the purpose of assessment is to find out whether a candidate possesses a particular broad ability (e.g. clinical skills) or a subset of abilities (e.g. history taking, physical examination, advising a patient) within a broad ability (e.g. clinical skills), then this would be analogous to a screening process for detecting a person with a clinical condition within a population. The purpose of the latter is to find out whether an individual is healthy (in relation to a given disease) or not, whereas the purpose of the former is to find out whether a candidate is competent (in relation to a particular ability) or not. How we set about finding whether an individual has or does not have a particular disease will provide us important insights into how assessment should be best planned and carried out. To complete this analogy, we will refer to some of the important steps of assessment that we explain in detail in the ensuing three chapters.

A good test knows what underlies the measurement

Let us take psychological stress as an example. Since it is an intangible concept, we should first have a theoretical conceptualisation of what 'psychological stress' entails, before we try to measure it. As it is intangible, direct assessment of stress is not possible. In educational assessment too, we assess abilities that are not overtly apparent and hence cannot be directly assessed, e.g. clinical reasoning, communication. These broad abilities or conceptual entities that define a person's ability are called 'constructs'.[1]

A good test picks up early warning signs or subtle changes of measurement

In the early stages of stress an individual may not recognise the symptoms and may not seek the help of a healthcare professional. This patient delay may lead to situations where stress has already led to considerable psychological damage. So, for efficient healthcare delivery early detection and prevention are more effective than cure. Screening tools therefore have to be able to pick up (or identify) individuals with early warning signs from the community. Hence, a screening test should be easily applied to all individuals in the community to distinguish those who have abnormal findings from those who do not. Similarly, no student will declare or even be aware at a summative assessment that he/she does not possess the required level of ability. Hence, a function of assessment is to identify the candidates who do not possess an appropriate level of the relevant construct.

A good test is known for its accuracy

Any tool that does not measure the construct of 'psychological stress' will not help us in identifying who is stressed. Hence, the tool that we select to measure stress should have a proven record (i.e. literature evidence) of measuring stress accurately. Similarly, in an educational setting, the assessment tool that we select to measure clinical reasoning, for example, should provide the examiners with an accurate measure of the candidate's clinical reasoning ability. This accuracy is called 'validity'. Validity is the ability or capacity of a test/examination tool to assess the construct that it is expected to assess.[2]

A good test uses a representative sample of content

Abstract and intangible constructs like psychological stress usually cannot be measured with a single magic measurement, such as a question that just asks the individual 'are you stressed?' Firstly, because individuals are relatively poor in self-assessment,[3] such overt questions are destined to fail in identifying those who are stressed. Secondly, constructs usually are multifaceted and cannot be simply measured from a single angle. Hence, we need to use a battery of questions about various situations, feelings and behaviours, such as 'how often you eat?', 'do you feel like eating?', 'do you bother to comb your hair?', 'at what time do you wake up every morning?', etc. A screening test with a battery of questions used to quantify how much of the construct (e.g. psychological stress) under measurement an individual has (e.g. psychological stress) is called a psychometric test or an inventory. Several questions rather than just one question is necessary to capture and assess every aspect of the construct so that the entire depth and breadth of the construct is captured. When we say 'captured' it goes without saying that no tool can capture every bit of or every facet of 'stress'. However, a cross section of all prominent behaviours, feelings and situations that represent everyday life would provide us a good enough picture of a person's stress level. As such, it is impossible and even undesirable for a screening tool to capture every facet of a person's life related to stress if its purpose is only to decide whether the person is stressed or not. However, an adequate 'sample' of instances as to how the person behaves, feels and thinks should provide a good enough measure of the person's stress level. In other words, the amount of data points or questions that we include in our screening tool should sufficiently inform us whether the person is stressed or not. The sample of questions that we select to include in the screening tool should represent (or cover) at least a segment of all possible major daily activities, situations and feelings. For example, we may not be able to include items on every meal that the individual takes or even items on breakfast, lunch and dinner separately, but a general question about meals should function as an adequate sample of the activities, thoughts, feelings related to meals. The adequacy of sampling should be such that the measure of stress we obtain with the questions that we include in the screening tool should be the same as (or very similar to) the measure that we would have obtained if we included every bit of the individual's daily life related to stress. This 'sufficient number of questions' in a screening tool for stress is the same as the sufficient number of items (or questions) included in an educational assessment to represent the construct under assessment, e.g. clinical reasoning. By including a sufficient distribution of items across the various aspects that adequately represent the construct that we want to measure, we support a type of validity known as 'content validity'.[4] Hence, the questions of an educational assessment must cover all the content areas that should be assessed, similar to items in the stress screening tool covering all major daily life events of a person. In educational assessment, we ensure that all content areas and learning outcomes that should be assessed are covered by a process called assessment blueprinting.[5]

A good test uses the right tools to measure the right content

Once the content of the items to quantify stress has been selected, these items will have to be accurately and precisely worded to convey the intended meaning unambiguously to the respondent. Hence, care should be taken when wording the items, so that all individuals will most likely interpret the same item the same way. Designing a good inventory that accurately assesses psychological stress will take several iterations and revisions in the wording. Then, the test will be also subjected to further piloting and validation, before being used to assess the stress levels of individuals. In educational assessment too, care should be exercised to word the questions precisely so that all candidates (and examiners) interpret the questions uniformly to extract the same meaning. If not, the said test would not assess the construct that the examiners intended to assess and hence cannot be claimed to assess the candidate ability validly.

A good test is pitched at the optimal level of difficulty

In life, some activities are often either easier or more difficult to recall than others. So, some items or questions in a screening tool may be more difficult to answer than the others, as a difficult item may be related to an activity that is difficult to recall (and hence to respond). A good screening tool should capture this natural variation of difficulty, rather than only containing overly easy or overly difficult items. Similarly, an educational test should capture the right level of difficulty that the construct under assessment is expected to assess, so that those who are successful at the test will be able to handle healthcare encounters to the expected professional level. We quantify the difficulty level of an assessment or assessment items by calculating an index called 'difficulty index' or 'facility index'.

A good test separates the haves from the have nots

If all items in a screening test for psychological stress are answered affirmatively by both those who have an unhealthy level of psychological stress and those who do not, the test will not be able to distinguish those who need healthcare support from those who don't. Hence, each item in the screening test should contribute to distinguishing or discriminating those who possess an abnormal level of the construct from those who do not. Without such discriminative ability, the individuals who are psychologically stressed and who are not, will end up with the same result or test score. Likewise, the questions or items of an educational assessment should contribute to separate or discriminate candidates who possess an adequate level of ability from those who don't. In educational jargon, this is called the discriminative ability (i.e. the ability to discriminate the incompetent from the competent) of an assessment. We calculate an index called 'discrimination index' to find out which tests or test items can separate the candidates who possess an adequate level of ability from those who do not possess the same adequate level of ability.

A good test is precise or error-free, as much as it can be

The items in the stress inventory should not only capture the entire construct of psychological stress comprehensively, but all items should only assess the said construct. As a result, the outcome of the assessment should be consistent over any number of administrations, so that an individual with a particular stress level will obtain the same score, if repeated. This is called 'reliability'. Often, reliability is measured by a measure of internal consistency such as Cronbach's alpha.[6] If the reliability is high, then the scale would measure the construct under measurement (i.e. psychological stress in this case) with minimal measurement error. If there is zero error (meaning the stress scale assesses nothing but psychological stress), then the reliability of the scale scores will be maximal or 1. If the scale measures everything other than psychological stress, then the error will be maximal (i.e. it is only the error that we would get out of the scale). Such an assessment would be totally unreliable. Usually, reliability will depend on the number of items in the measuring tool — and generally, higher the number of items, higher the reliability. The same is true for educational assessment. All assessment questions should assess the same construct under assessment as precisely as possible. If so, there would be a minimal error within the test score. If there is zero error, then a candidate's test score should represent entirely the ability of the candidate. As in a health screening tool, higher the number of items or questions, higher would be the reliability of the test score. Usually, a reliability of 0.8 or above is considered acceptable.

A good test employs the right method and the right measurers

If self-assessment is not valid, then we could employ trained professionals to observe an individual's behaviours to identify who is stressed and who is not. Since the observer will have to observe a behaviour or an activity and then make an interpretation as to whether it is within the accepted range of behaviour or not, such decisions can contain an element of misinterpretation or an element of error. So, the observers should be trained to detect (i.e. observe, interpret and categorise) various behaviours of a person. For the accurate detection of a person who needs healthcare attention related to stress, we must depend on more than one trained observer. Training of observers or raters should be targeted at minimising the raters' consideration of extraneous factors (e.g. dress, speaking style) when rating a subject. Due to the logistics involved, observation is not implemented routinely for screening purposes. Rather, in healthcare, whenever possible, we use more cost-effective tools such as inventories for psychological stress, for screening purposes. However, assessment of skills in an educational setting cannot be performed credibly using an inventory-type written assessment. Hence, observation is essential in skills assessment in education. Such assessment information must be collected using multiple observers, for the same reasons given above for using multiple observers to identify a person under stress, precisely and accurately.

A good test collates and interprets many measurements appropriately

Since whether an individual is stressed or not cannot be decided using one item, several items are used. This is so, whether it is an inventory-based assessment or observable assessment using rating scales. In the latter, there will be several ratings assessing the different aspects of stress-related behaviour, e.g. calmness, approach to a situation, etc. The scores of all these items should be put together (e.g. usually added) to produce a composite score, where such a score is meaningful. Similarly, where indicated, the scores for all the questions or items of an assessment are generally collated (usually by adding the score for all the items/questions) to obtain a comprehensive picture of the candidate ability.

Next in stress assessment, the total score that an individual scored (using either an inventory or an observer rating) should be interpreted to determine whether the stress score is high enough to identify (or diagnose) that he/she is stressed to an unhealthy level. This is usually done by carrying out validation studies to determine the score range that normal individuals in the society would score, using some external gold standard. Any score above this normal range is considered as a stress level that would compromise health. In an educational assessment, likewise, we ask whether a particular test score indicates a level of ability that could be deemed adequate to be a safe practitioner. This level of adequacy is determined by a process of standard setting to determine the pass mark. Yet, a fundamental difference is that in educational assessment there is rarely a validated external gold standard. Therefore, any cut-off score is based on a collation of expert judgements using one of the many available standard setting methods.[7,8]

A good test is followed by appropriate feedback and remediation

Once the individuals with high stress levels have been identified, they will be attended to in a one-to-one health professional–patient encounter, e.g. a patient in a clinic with a doctor. This encounter would involve more qualitative, deep analysis of the individual's stress levels and reasons for the same, in a personalised manner. Similarly, once the failing candidates are identified they should be remediated one-to-one with constructive feedback from a suitable mentor/teacher. Here, unlike in screening, one need not collect snapshot data from many observers/teachers as the attention provided is more individualised. Rather, it is more a qualitative, continuing, one-to-one relationship.

The foregoing, using psychological stress as an example, shows how close (if not the same) the rationale of screening in clinical practice is to educational assessment. It is not only psychological stress, any clinical process that spans from patient identification (i.e. screening) to treatment could be compared with the educational practice from identifying students with less than the desired ability to remediation. To illustrate that this analogy is not unique to psychological stress, another comparison using the 'measurement of blood pressure' as the example is summarised in Table 1.

Table 1. A comparison of the rationale of the process of measuring blood pressure with the process of educational assessment.

Measurement property	Measurement of blood pressure	Educational assessment
Purpose	The purpose (more often than not) is to screen presumably healthy individuals to find out whether a person's blood pressure is appropriate for his age and other sociodemographic characteristics	The purpose is to find out whether the candidates have an appropriate level of ability for their level of training
Construct	Blood pressure, the construct under measurement, is a concept that is intangible	Ability of a candidate, the construct under assessment, is an intangible concept

(Continued)

Table 1. (*Continued*)

Measurement property	Measurement of blood pressure	Educational assessment
Instrument of measurement	An appropriate instrument to measure blood pressure (i.e. the construct) should be selected, e.g. a sphygmomanometer rather than a barometer	An appropriate educational assessment that will provide information on the construct that is measured should be selected, e.g. Objective Structured Clinical Examination (OSCE), rather than multiple choice questions (MCQ), to assess the psychomotor domain
Content validity	All components of the construct (i.e. both systolic and diastolic blood pressure) rather than a part of it (e.g. systolic blood pressure only) should be identified for measurement. Also, the measurement may have to include the blood pressure in certain postures, e.g. sitting, standing and reclining positions	The educational tool should ideally capture every part of what is intended to measure (i.e. construct). If every part is logistically not possible, then an appropriate sample of the components should be selected to comprehensively represent the construct. This is done through blueprinting
Validity of measurement	Correct procedure should be followed (e.g. person in resting state, a calibrated sphygmomanometer, correct cuff size, correct Korotkoff sound, etc.)	Correct construction of the test items is needed to capture the construct accurately, e.g. following MCQ writing guidelines.
Reliability	Measuring blood pressure just once will not provide with a precise measure due to physiological variation and measurement (e.g. operator, instrument) error. Hence, the measurement should be carried out a number of times to arrive at a measurement with the least error	Assessing with just one examiner (in skills or attitude assessment) or assessing only with a few items (in knowledge, skills or attitude assessment) will not provide a stable result due to variation in candidate performance in different assessment situations, examiner error, etc.

Table 1. (*Continued*)

Measurement property	Measurement of blood pressure	Educational assessment
Difficulty of items	All blood pressure measurements are not expected to provide the same result, e.g. standing, sitting, reclining blood pressure will be different	All items/questions are not expected to produce same score. Easy questions will produce higher scores and difficult questions will produce lower scores
Discrimination of items	A certain unique blood pressure measurement (e.g. blood pressure in the reclining position) will enable the separation of patients with certain conditions (e.g. postural hypotension) from the others	A certain item/question of an assessment will enable the separation or discrimination of candidates, who possess more of the ability (or a subset of the ability) that this item assesses, from the other candidates
Collation of results	The blood pressure readings taken in different instances of a person will have to be put together in a certain logical way, e.g. average systolic blood pressure in the sitting position	The scores of a candidate in different items/questions will have to be aggregated in a logical way, e.g. total score of items that assessed a particular sub-ability/learning outcome
Interpretation of the result	Values of a normal, healthy person in the reference age group of the person under measurement are needed to decide whether the blood pressure, representing all the readings collected, is within the healthy limits are not	The acceptable overall score (based on the candidate scoring in all assessment items representing a particular ability) of a candidate is compared with the minimum level of ability expected. This minimum level identified is the pass mark calculated using an appropriate standard setting process
Feedback and remedial process	Those persons (i.e. patients) identified with abnormal blood pressure levels will need to go through further intense and in-depth investigations with a suitably qualified health	The candidate who scored below the pass mark will require further investigation to find out why they scored less in certain items. Then, depending on the areas covered by these low

(*Continued*)

Table 1. (*Continued*)

Measurement property	Measurement of blood pressure	Educational assessment
	professional to identify the cause and then undergo appropriate treatment. All other persons could be assured that their blood pressure is within normal limits	scoring items, individualised feedback should be given by an educational supervisor/mentor. All other candidates should be congratulated as their overall ability level is above the level expected, but they should be informed if they need improvement in certain areas that they may have shown a relative weakness

The above examples go on to inform us that good practices in educational assessment are not unique to education, but common to clinical practice and perhaps many other practices. These practices have stood the test of time within many spheres of life. Also, they can be readily justified both theoretically and empirically. It is our hope that you will better understand and appreciate the 'what', 'why' and 'how' that you will read in Chapters 1–3, using the rationale provided in this introduction.

Chapter 1: Assess Why?

In the scenario at the beginning of this section, one can ask whether the graduates aren't right. When they have been successful at the medical school assessments, they can naturally expect their communication and procedural skills (along with the other competencies) to be up to the expected standard for them to be safe practitioners. So, notwithstanding their inadequacies in the expected competencies, the graduates' understanding about the expected role of assessment in medical school seems to be correct: assessments are to be passed only by the candidates who have achieved the minimum level of ability to make them safe healthcare professionals. Hence, a primary purpose of assessment in the medical school is to identify and certify those candidates who are safe for practice. This is perhaps the commonest and the most important overall reason why we assess.

However, for the medical school to identify and graduate only those who are safe for practice (i.e. are competent or have achieved all the competencies), the school must put in place a battery of assessments that serve a variety of purposes. These purposes can be primarily categorised into two major groups: formative assessment and summative assessment.

A. Formative Assessment

If a school wants most (if not all) of its students to graduate as competent healthcare professionals, then the school must inform them periodically on how well they have progressed thus far in their journey towards achieving all the required competencies. For this reason, the school must implement a series of assessments, not necessarily only to decide who passes and who fails, but to inform the candidates about their strengths and weaknesses. Since these assessments are used to improve learning, they are called formative assessment.

Assessment for learning and formative assessment are quite similar in that they provide information-rich feedback to the student for improving their learning. However, one important difference is that in assessment for learning the student is required to make use of the feedback to achieve the requirements of a given stage of learning, but in formative assessment it is left to the student to choose whether or not to use the feedback.

Based on these assessment results, the candidates can identify the areas that they are weak in and take corrective measures. However, students may not always be good at identifying their own weaknesses.[3] Hence, feedback by teachers in conjunction with self-assessment by the student offers richer information for improvement. Additionally, reflecting on the differences between the various sources of feedback (e.g. self versus others) enables the student to sharpen their self-assessment skills.

Also, both the learners and the teachers can use the results of formative assessment to monitor and profile the progress of the learners. Thus, an important function of formative assessment is to support learning.

Although formative assessment is said to be for the benefit of the candidate, other stakeholders (e.g. examination boards, teachers, institutions) could also benefit from such assessment by finding out whether the students have learnt what they were supposed to learn. Progress testing is an example of this type of assessment. In progress testing, all students, irrespective of their level of training (i.e. year of study) take the same assessment pitched at the exit level, every year. The expectation is as the students' progress in the curriculum, their assessment scores will also progressively increase. A significant proportion of students not meeting this expectation signals a warning to the above stakeholders to initiate remedial measures.

B. Summative Assessment

Since patient safety is too important an issue to be left for the students alone to auto-correct themselves based on the feedback on their assessment results, a health professions school by design would not allow a candidate to progress to the next stage/phase of learning within the curriculum, if the student does not show the required level of achievement. To decide whether they possess the required level of ability, health professions schools conduct assessments that could provide trustworthy and dependable (or accurate and precise) information about the candidate's ability. If a candidate passes these assessments, she is allowed to proceed to the next stage in the curriculum; if she fails, she is not. These assessments provide information to take important pass/fail decisions that will affect the candidate's career. So, they are high stakes tests and are generally referred to as 'summative assessment'. As the primary focus of summative assessment is the determination of the level of ability (i.e. the determination of the level of learning) of the candidate these assessments are also called 'assessment of learning'.

Assessment of learning can take many different forms. Sometimes, assessment of learning is for the award of distinctions, medals and other merit awards. These assessments by their very nature are conducted not to decide whether the candidate has achieved a basic required standard. Instead, they are conducted to find out who is/are worthy of special recognition among a group of top performers. Thus, it is a ranking exercise. Hence, ideally, there should be separate tailor-made assessments to award merit. However, due to resource constraints, at least some institutions use the same assessment both to decide who passes and who receives merit. One could argue that this is not an optimal compromise, as the difficulty level of the content and the constructs (or broad underlying abilities) that should be assessed in these two instances would be significantly different.

Selection of candidates to be admitted to a particular course could also be considered as a form of assessment of learning. In this case, the abilities assessed are those that the candidates have acquired in their past learning, rather than within a particular course. Here too, ranking of candidates might be the focus.

The assessments conducted for the admission to professional societies or associations could also be considered a variation of selection tests and can be categorised as assessment of learning. The content and abilities assessed in this instance would be to determine the worthiness of the candidate to be admitted to a particular professional body.

C. Other Uses of Assessment Data

Sometimes, assessments are conducted for special reasons. Or else, as is more often the case, the existing assessments are used for certain unconventional purposes. Occasionally, there may be assessments held for quality assurance and accreditation purposes of curricula and study programmes. Such assessments are high stakes for the institutions. Hence, for the institution, these assessments are summative in nature. However, for the candidates, they would mostly fulfil a formative function.

D. The Summative versus Formative Dilemma

From the foregoing it is clear that formative assessment aims to ensure competent graduates by driving the learning process, whereas summative assessment aims to ensure competent graduates by measuring the level of competence. Another difference is the way both approaches try to direct student learning. Summative assessment drives learning in a more behaviourist way, with failure or success on the test acting as punishment or reward. Formative assessment, on the other hand, seeks to drive learning in a more constructivist way by making the student derive meaning out of feedback and assume agency for their own learning. In practice, however, many assessments fulfil both these functions to a lesser or greater degree. Often, partly due to this overlap in assessment practice, the two purposes are commonly confused. Following are two of the commonest such misconceptions about summative and formative assessment.

(a) *Misconception 1: If scores or grades are awarded, they are summative tests and if scores or grades are not awarded, they are formative tests.*

The presence of assessment scores or grades does not necessarily make an assessment summative. This is especially so if those marks are not considered for pass/fail decisions. Similarly, in rare instances, a panel of examiners may decide whether a candidate has passed or failed by merely observing the candidate performance or by merely reading the candidate's answer, without awarding any scores or grades. So, the presence or absence of test scores or grades does not automatically qualify an assessment to be labelled summative or formative. Rather, one should find out the purpose of the test before deciding whether the assessment is formative or summative.

(b) *Misconception 2: When an assessment is followed by feedback it is a formative assessment, and when there is no feedback it is summative.*

It is true that feedback is a core feature of formative assessment. However, that does not prohibit summative assessments from giving feedback. In fact, feedback should be sound educational practice for any assessment, be it formative or summative.

So, one of the main reasons for the summative and formative confusion is trying to label assessment without clearly identifying the purpose of assessment.

Apart from the above confusions, the divide between formative and summative assessment may not be clear-cut due to the intrinsic characteristics of a given assessment. We argue that it need not be clear-cut either. Ideally, all assessment would have a formative function. This means, at least the failing candidates should know why they failed. However, even the passing candidates should be informed about their relative strengths and weaknesses.

Similarly, predominantly formative assessments sometimes may assume summative roles. It is common practice, at least in certain schools, to carry forward a small percentage of marks of all or some of its predominantly formative continuous assessments to contribute to the final score of a given course, module or unit within the curriculum. This happens due to a gamut of pragmatic reasons, such as:

1. Sometimes there are complaints that the students do not take formative assessment seriously if some summative role is not built into it. This is an example of 'assessment drives learning'.

2. By spreading the number of assessments over the duration of the course, the students could collect marks at different points within the assessment system. This will relieve the exam stress as the students would then be aware that the final assessment would not be as high stakes as it would be, since a certain percentage of this high stakes final assessment score has been already secured by the candidate.

3. The curriculum is too broad to be sampled adequately within a single end-of-course summative assessment. Hence, the continuous assessments have to be used to fulfil a summative function. Since they are continuous assessments, the students also get an opportunity to test their ability midway in the course and then take corrective measures to overcome their weaknesses, as identified by these continuous assessments. The latter is the formative function of such continuous assessment.

4. Usually, the curriculum needs to be achieved in stages, and the ability in each stage is a prerequisite to move to the next. Hence, the continuous assessment held at each stage of the course needs to be used for the summative function of deciding who could proceed to the next stage of the course. As seen above, these continuous assessments also fulfil a formative function as their results offer the candidates an opportunity to take corrective measures with regard to their weaknesses.

5. Assessments are costly. To implement purely formative continuous assessment and then conduct another set of summative assessments may be too resource intensive.

Some may argue that in the above instances, the continuous assessments are summative rather than formative. This argument is not invalid. However, if the main purpose of the assessment is feedback, then some may also argue that based on its predominant function, it is fairer to call this type of assessment formative. If, however, the purpose of the continuous assessment is to sample the curriculum more broadly to supplement an end-of-course summative assessment, then the primary purpose behind these assessments is summative. Such assessments, based on their predominant purpose, are justified being considered as summative assessment. In summary, this discussion makes it clear that rarely will an assessment be purely formative or purely summative and, in most instances, there is a combination of aims. It is important that the assessment design must therefore be deliberate and purposeful with these aims and how they are combined.

Therefore, we argue that it is best that these dual-purpose assessments are detailed more elaborately, rather than simply labelling them summative or formative. For example, in the latter instance above, where the main purpose of assessment is to sample the curriculum, this continuous assessment is best described as 'a summative assessment with formative features'. Alternatively, a continuous assessment that is primarily carried out to provide feedback, although a small percentage of it contributes to the final assessment score, could be described as 'a formative assessment with summative features'.

Hence, from a pragmatic standpoint, instituting predominantly formative assessment with a relatively small summative function is not necessarily wrong, provided that the distinct summative and formative roles are clear to all stakeholders. Also, as we would discuss in Chapter 3 of this section, in programmatic assessment,[9] the summative and formative distinction is not used anymore, but instead all assessment contributes to both optimising feedback and enhancing the quality of decision-making on students' progress.

Finally, before we end this discussion on formative and summative assessment, it should be cautioned that there are also dangers in mixing the formative and summative functions. As we will discuss in Chapter 3, the summative function could easily engulf the formative function, if the candidates attempt to hide their weaknesses in order to score more and thereby losing an opportunity to rectifying their weaknesses. So, mixing of formative and summative functions needs to be done with caution. One way to exercise such caution is to broadly divide the assessment of a candidate into two parts: scoring the candidate performance and interpretation of the score. When scoring the candidate performance, it is best that the scorers (examiners) do not consider formative and summative roles of assessment. Once the scoring is completed, however, the formative and summative functions could be considered for the interpretation of scores. In short, the assessment process (i.e. scoring the candidate) and the different ways of using the results of such a process should be kept separate.

E. Summary

Based on the purpose of assessment, the reasons for assessment could be broadly divided into formative and summative functions. Other purposes of carrying out assessments such as progress tests serve a formative function to both the students and the institution. Some others, such as to award merit, to select suitable applicants to a course, to admit members to a professional body, college or society, are mainly variants of the summative function of assessment. If assessments are carried out solely for the purposes of quality assurance and accreditation, they could be considered as summative for the institution, but formative for the students.

In practice, however, due to both logistical (e.g. resource constraints) and educational (e.g. to encourage and support student learning) reasons the same assessment could serve both formative and summative functions. Such blurring of the formative and summative boundaries is acceptable as long as all the stakeholders are aware of the dual purposes of the same assessment. Programmatic assessment is a clear example of all assessments being considered both summative and formative. However, one needs to be careful to avoid undue tension between summative and formative functions within the same assessment. If not, students will focus on the summative functions of the assessment at the expense of its formative benefits. Hence, the mixing of formative and summative functions needs to be handled with utmost care and caution.

Chapter 2: Assess What?

In the scenario at the beginning of this section, the graduates claimed that they had passed all examinations in both communication skills and procedural skills. In that case, one pertinent question to ask is what was assessed in communication skills and procedural skills. Did the content in these examinations actually capture the required aspects necessary to practise communication skills and procedural skills? For example, if the assessment was only on communication with adults, then the graduates may struggle communicating with children, as their ability of communicating with children would be unknown to the examination board that certified their competence. The assumption that communicating with adults makes one automatically proficient in communicating with children defies the tenets of context specificity.[10] If the assessment did capture the right aspects, then did it include an adequate amount of assessment material to represent each of the aspects related to communication skills and procedural skills? These are all concerns related to how valid the content is. Hence, these questions would evaluate the content validity of the assessment concerned.

Guion[4] stated that if content-based inferences of test scores are to be meaningful, the observed performances should: 1. be a representative sample from the domain that is intended to be assessed; 2. be assessed appropriately; and 3. constitute a sample large enough to control sampling error . Below, we discuss 1 and 3 of the above stipulations. As 2 essentially means 'how to assess' it will be covered in Chapter 3.

A. Representativeness of the Assessment

Ideally, we should assess the entire curriculum. However, logistics and resources do not allow us to assess all that has been taught, i.e. the entire curriculum. Most medical curricula span several years, whereas the assessments are reduced to a few hours. So, the fundamental problem with any assessment is that we have a large curriculum and a comparatively small examination. Hence, much of the content within a curriculum will not be summatively assessed during any examination or even in a series of examinations. However, often the intent of an examination is to find out the level of ability of a candidate in relation to the entire curriculum. *How can we bridge the gap between the intent of assessing the entire curriculum and actually (due to practical constraints) assessing only a part of the curriculum?* This is the most fundamental question that any assessment should satisfactorily answer. The better one answers this fundamental question, the better one can design assessments and interpret test scores.

This problem is very similar (if not the same) to a problem that we come across in research. In research, the research question that we usually investigate is in relation to an entire *population*. For example, what is the average systolic blood pressure of adult males in a particular geographical location, e.g. in one country? If this is the research question that we want to investigate, then the best option that we have is to measure systolic blood pressure of every male in that country and then use all these measurements to compute the mean systolic blood pressure. This is analogous to assessing the entire curriculum at an examination, i.e. the entire curriculum is analogous to the population of adult males in the country concerned. However, we all know that measuring the blood pressure of every male in a country is very resource-draining and hence, unfeasible. So, the alternative approach that we adopt is we take a *sample* of adult males from this population to measure the blood pressure. If our sample represents the population, then the mean blood pressure that we compute using the sample will be very close (if not the same) to the mean that we would have computed had we measured the blood pressure of the entire population. The same principle can be applied to resolve the most fundamental problem that we have in any assessment, i.e. how to deal with a large curriculum with a comparatively small examination. In this case, the curriculum is the population and the assessment is the sample. However, for this ploy to deliver a desirable result (i.e. for the overall score that we award a candidate in an assessment to be very similar, if not the same, to the score that we would have awarded even if we assessed the entire curriculum) the curriculum content should be well represented in the assessment — just like the sample should represent the population for the conclusions that we derive from the sample to be valid. Hence, if any assessment is a 'representative' sample of the curriculum, then such an assessment could be used with sufficient content validity to derive conclusions about the candidate's ability on the curriculum. If not, the validity of our conclusions can only be confined to that particular assessment and not the entire curriculum.

How can we obtain a representative sample from the curriculum, when we are developing an assessment? The first step is to realise that a curriculum is made up of content areas (i.e. the subject matter) and learning outcomes (i.e. the intended broad abilities or constructs that the learner needs to achieve by learning the content or subject matter). For example, a module on the cardiovascular system or a lesson on congestive cardiac failure could be considered as a content element, depending on how large or small (i.e. the granularity of) the content area that one wants to define. Similarly, communication skills can be considered as a learning outcome. When designing an assessment, we need to sample the curriculum content and learning outcomes in such a way that all the curriculum content areas and all learning outcomes are represented in our assessment. The framework that we use to ensure that each learning outcome and each curriculum content are represented in the assessment is called an assessment blueprint.[5] Some in mainstream education call it 'table of specifications'.[11]

An assessment blueprint is a table that conventionally (but not necessarily) contains the learning outcomes in columns and the curriculum content in rows (Table 2). All the cells in the blueprint should, in general, map the entire curriculum. The only exception to this may be a few cells, which represent a few content areas that do not address a particular learning outcome. For example, there could be an entirely theory-based module or a lesson that does not address any procedural skills. However, such cells in the blueprint should be relatively few and far between, and they could be blocked out to indicate that these cells are not expected to be part of the blueprint.

A tick in the assessment blueprint in Table 2 denotes a question (or item) to represent a particular learning outcome and a curriculum content. When selecting assessment material (i.e. questions) using the blueprint, the assessment developer (i.e. the assessment committee or the examination board) should ensure that sufficient assessment items (e.g. questions, stations, cases) are included to represent each column and each row. At the same time, the selection of questions should ensure that there is at least one tick in each column and each row, for the assessment to be a representative sample of the curriculum. It should also be stated

Table 2. An illustration of a model assessment blueprint.

	Competency 1 e.g. clinical skills	Competency 2 e.g. communication skills	Competency 3	Competency 4	…	Competency n	Total
Content area 1 e.g. cardio vascular system	✓	–	✓	–	–	✓	–
Content area 2 e.g. endocrine system	–	✓	–	✓	–	–	–
Content area 3	✓	✓	–	–	–	✓	–
… … …	–	–	–	–	–	–	–
Content area n	✓	✓	–	✓	–	✓	–
Total	–	–	–	–	–	–	–

that each cell (i.e. the intersection of a particular learning outcome and a particular content area) within the blueprint could contain more than one tick or one item. If a particular cell is considered more important, then such a cell could be represented in the assessment by more than one item/question. However, selecting more than one item to represent a particular cell has an opportunity cost, i.e. including more than one item within a cell would be at the expense of representing another cell of the blueprint and hence representing another unique combination of a content area and a learning outcome in the assessment.

When selecting items, it is important to note that an item (or a tick in the blueprint) should represent not just a question or the instructions to the candidate, but the expected answer or the expected behaviour by the candidate. This is because it is not the items (or questions) but the curriculum material (i.e. content areas and learning outcomes) that should be sampled by the blueprint. So, by including items in the blueprint, we actually accept that those items are part of a representative sample of the curriculum that they test, i.e. the expected answer or the behaviour to the said items.

It should also be stated here that this is the simplest form of assessment blueprint that one could think of. A blueprint could be more complex if one wants to sample curriculum dimensions other than the learning outcomes and content. For example, in the scenario that we discussed at the beginning of this section, if the examination board wants to assure that the candidates are proficient in communication skills related to not only adult patients but also paediatric patients, then for each content area (e.g. congestive cardiac failure) there could be two sub-rows representing adult and paediatric age groups. Alternatively, the same information could be included as two sub-columns under communication skills to represent the two age groups. One word of caution though about developing highly complex assessment blueprints. Subdivision of columns and rows into too many sub-dimensions poses special challenges to achieve examiner consensus on item classification.[12] So, it is crucial that the examination boards decide on the essential, few sub-dimensions that would come under learning outcomes and contents, if they want to sample on aspects other than curriculum content and learning outcomes.

The categorisation of items/questions into different rows and different columns in the blueprint should ideally be done through consensus among the members of the examination board. However, if an examination board wants to validate the blueprint, then an index called 'content validity index' (CVI) could be computed.[13] A CVI should ideally be created for each item/question, by a group of experts, who would rate how appropriate each item is to be categorised in a given row and a column. This rating is usually done on a 3–5 scale, where the maximum rating point (i.e. category) of the scale indicates absolute agreement with the positioning of the item within blueprint and the minimum rating indicates the opposite. Then, the proportion of experts who agrees (i.e. rates either 4 or 5 on a typical 5-point scale) on an item's positioning in a particular cell is calculated. This is the CVI. Ideally, a CVI of more than 0.8 (i.e. 80% of the members of the examination board deciding that a particular item is appropriately positioned in the blueprint) is considered sufficient validation of an item's positioning in the blueprint. If an item appears in more than one cell, then there could be more than one CVI per item, each corresponding to the cell that the said item appears in the blueprint.

Alternatively, members of such a panel could be asked to provide a narrative explanation as to why a particular item is relevant and valid for the domain to be tested. Typically, such narratives would have to surpass motherhood statements such as 'essential knowledge' or 'this is just basic knowledge'. Narratives can be constructed around risk to patients, incidence and prevalence, relevance of the item in relation to larger concepts, etc. Both the quantitative and qualitative approaches have their pros and cons. Quantitative approaches are easier to explain and perform, but generally require larger panels to achieve sufficient reliability of judgements, whereas qualitative approaches are more difficult to explain and more time-consuming.

It is readily understandable from the above description of the blueprinting process that blueprinting follows a particular type of sampling, called stratified sampling. The curriculum is stratified into learning outcomes and content areas and the sampling is carried out in such a way to ensure that each of the strata (i.e. layers denoting learning outcomes and content) is represented in the assessment or the sample. A pertinent question then would be 'why stratified sampling'? Or 'why not simple random sampling'? For instance, it is well known that simple random sampling is the best sampling strategy as it offers an equal probability for every item in the population (or curriculum) to be selected to the sample (or the examination). Also, simple random sampling would account for all possible classifications (or dimensions) in the population (e.g. age [adult-paediatric], gender, content, learning outcomes), rather than the two or three classifications considered in the stratification process. If so, why stratified sampling instead of random sampling?

The reason for using a stratified sampling strategy in assessment blueprinting has much to do with the number of items (i.e. questions) that could be included in the sample (i.e. assessment). Stratified sampling is preferred in blueprinting because of the relatively few items (i.e. questions) that we could include in the sample (i.e. assessment). For simple random sampling to work well a large sample size is a must. Using simple random sampling to select a very small sample size runs the risk of selecting a non-representative sample, i.e. examination material missing out on certain content areas and learning outcomes. Hence, we use stratified sampling in blueprinting as we need to select items (i.e. questions) perforce to represent the various important strata in the population (i.e. curriculum).

B. Adequacy of the Assessment

This brings us to the important issue of how many items are necessary for the items to represent the curriculum. There are two important aspects to consider in this respect: 1. adequacy of the total number of items/questions and 2. adequacy of the number of items within a particular layer in the blueprint.

1. *Adequacy of the total number of items/questions*

If the members of the examination board (or an expert panel of examiners) concur that the number of items included in the blueprint is adequate and adding another item does not offer a significant increase of additional information about the candidate ability, then this should be the point at which the sampling of items should cease. This is similar to the point of data saturation that indicates the termination of recruiting participants in qualitative research. It is also comparable to a standard diagnostic procedure. When a clinician is satisfied that he or she has gathered enough diagnostic information to make a full diagnosis and understand the whole patient problem there is no need for further additional diagnostic procedures. Such a 'saturation of information' approach is defensible as long as the judgement on saturation is made by people with sufficient expertise to arrive at such an informed judgement. Therefore, the assumption underlying this approach is that the members of the examination board have a good and comprehensive overview on the requirements of the curriculum.

Alternatively, in quantitative research, we use formulae to estimate the sample size necessary to produce a conclusive result, i.e. a result that could be relied upon or a result that will not change from sample to sample or a conclusion, which is generalisable beyond the sample. In assessment too, it is possible to use past results to carry out decision studies using generalisability theory or classical test theory (i.e. Spearman–Brown prophecies) to estimate the number of items and/or the number examiners (in the case of skills assessment) required to produce a generalisable result. The adequacy of the number of items could be more concretely validated by post-assessment reliability studies. This means that the total number of ticks in the above blueprint should not only represent all columns and all rows, but should be in total sufficient to generate a generalisable (i.e. reliable) overall candidate result as well. As this quantitative analysis is essentially a reliability analysis, it illustrates the intrinsic link between reliability and validity. Hence the reason for considering reliability evidence as legitimate evidence to support validity by contemporary theories of validity.[14]

2. *Adequacy of the number of items within a particular layer in the blueprint*

When all that we have discussed so far has been ensured, we may now be in a situation where all rows and columns of the blueprint are covered and the total number of items (or the number of ticks in the blueprint) is adequate, but still the number of items (or the ticks) within a particular row or column in the blueprint is too low or too high, i.e. under- or over-representation of a row or a column in the blueprint. So, this refers to an imbalance of the relative representation within columns and rows. Such imbalances are best resolved through discussion among the examiners or members of the examination board before the finalisation of the blueprint. To aid such a discussion two strategies could be useful.

First, the blueprint displaying the total selected items (i.e. the total number of ticks) within each row and each column would be useful. It is important to note here that the totals of each of the rows and columns need not be the same. Some rows and columns of the blueprint could be sampled more, depending on the volume and importance of the aspect represented by the said column or row within the curriculum. A rational way of determining the weightings apportioned to each row and each column would be to weight each item (or each tick) based on the maximum score that each item carries, before computing the row and column totals.

Second, a CVI could be created for each row and each column by requesting the members of the examination board (i.e. experts) to rate whether the content representation (i.e. the number of ticks) within a column or a row is adequate, on a scale similar to that described previously. Then the proportion of examiners who provided a rating that confirmed the adequacy of the number of items should be calculated for each row and each column. A CVI of more than 0.8 should be considered as a confirmation of the adequacy of the number of items to represent a given column or row.

C. How Valid is Content Validity?

Content validity is somewhat a disputed term, at least historically. If validity is 'the degree to which evidence and theory support the interpretations of test scores entailed by proposed uses of tests',[15] then content validity could be defined as 'the degree to which the evidence and theory related to test content support the interpretation of test scores given the intended purposes of the test'. The controversy lies in the non-use of 'interpretation of test scores' as evidence to validate the content of a test when evaluating content validity. For example, Sireci[16] claimed that content validity deals with test domain definition, domain representation, domain relevance and appropriateness of the test development process. This exposition of content validity, however, does not provide any relationship of content with the interpretation of scores.[17] So, the roots of this controversy about 'content validity' stem from the non-involvement of test scores in the validation of content. Quoting Cronbach[18] and Messick,[19] Guion[4] aptly summarised this controversy as 'validity of any sort is an attribute of scores rather than the tests themselves'. However, at least at that time, content validity was viewed as a 'sort' of validity of 'tests themselves', thus dissociating it (i.e. content validity) from the scores.

Kane[20] proposed a plausible compromise to this controversy by positing that although for direct measurement of holistic performance (e.g. playing a piano or hand washing in clinical practice) the behaviour itself would be sufficient to determine the ability of the candidate, i.e. by interpreting the test scores of such holistic behaviour. However, we assess competence measures that are mostly indirect. In assessment we can only observe behaviour; even ticking boxes in a multiple-choice examination is behaviour, but we seek to infer from that behaviour cognitive abilities or mental activities. These cognitive abilities or mental abilities cannot be observed directly and therefore have to be inferred from behaviour of verbalisation. For such indirect measurements of ability such as those that combine multiple fragmented pieces of ability (e.g. written MCQ tests, some OSCE stations) to construct a clear enough 'picture' of candidate ability, content coverage by the test (i.e. content validity) is an important consideration when interpreting test scores. Why direct observation of holistic tasks would be adequate in itself to cover all the content is because the behaviour in holistic (as opposed to fragmented) tasks cannot be carried out without completing all the content or all the steps of the task. Hence, all the content pertaining to the said task will have to be tested. For example, all the steps of hand washing are needed to perform hand washing successfully and hence these steps will automatically be tested in a test of hand washing. If the steps of hand washing are sampled, the candidate will not be able to perform the act of hand washing.

Validity based on interpretative arguments which Kane[21] later proposed, drawing on Cronbach's[22] (p. 103) famous quote that 'a proposition deserves some degree of trust only when it has survived serious attempts to falsify it', further underscores the importance of test content. This is so, as generalisation of test scores beyond the test material (or content) is one key argument for which Kane[21] recommends seeking interpretative evidence. Interpreting test scores beyond the test content calls for test material or content to represent a larger domain or construct of measurement. The most important corollary of this is that a test is never valid per se but always valid for a certain purpose or inference. For example, if the candidate's scores in handwashing are interpreted to estimate the candidate ability's in scrubbing, then the domain of handwashing is expanded beyond the simple act of handwashing that the examiner would have observed before scoring the candidate. If so, only using the scores of handwashing may constitute inadequate evidence, if at all, to estimate a candidate's ability in scrubbing. The reason for this is scrubbing has steps that handwashing does not test, i.e. steps (or content) of handwashing and scrubbing are not similar enough to extend the interpretation of handwashing scores to cover scrubbing. Such an interpretative approach to content validity is further supported by the aforementioned Standards for Educational and Psychological Testing,[15] where content is considered as one of the five core evidence sources fundamental to the appropriate interpretation of test scores. These five evidence sources are: test content; response formats; internal structure of the test; relationship of test scores with other variables; and testing consequences.

D. Summary

Assessment of 'what' is mainly concerned with the appropriateness, the representativeness and the adequacy of the assessment content considered to support the interpretation of test scores. The appropriateness and the representativeness of the content should be determined by a group of experts prior to the assessment, using tools such as the assessment blueprint and the CVI. The overall adequacy of the content included in the assessment should be determined by both expert consensus and reliability studies. The adequacy of each competency and each content area assessed could be verified by scrutinising the row and column totals in the blueprint by either a group of experts or calculating a CVI for each column and each row.

Although content validity is a term that has generated much debate and controversy, there is little doubt that the quality and adequacy of the content included in any assessment should be subjected to strict quality control. Such quality control of the assessment content assumes even greater importance when one considers that the evidence of content validity, as described in this chapter, is perhaps one of the few forms of evidence that can be controlled by an examination board prior to administering the examination. Most other forms of evidence to support validity would only be available after the examination, i.e. when the examination results are available.

Chapter 3: Assess How?

Let us go back to the scenario at the beginning of this section. What could be the reason for graduates passing all the assessments but being incompetent in certain abilities? Could it not be due to the use of an invalid assessment method? For example, if communication skills and procedural skills were assessed by written assessment, then would such assessment validly assess the graduates' ability in communication and clinical procedures? In this chapter, we discuss how assessment should be selected, constructed, delivered and interpreted, so that outcomes such as those mentioned in the aforesaid scenario can be avoided.

A. How Should Assessment Be Selected?

The selection of an assessment method should be dictated mainly by what needs to be assessed. Miller's pyramid[23] can be used as a simple guide to selecting an appropriate assessment method (Fig. 1).

The first step in selecting the most appropriate assessment would be to find out the 'level of assessment', according to the Miller's pyramid. As shown by the example at the beginning of this section, if the intention (what needs to be assessed) is to assess the candidates' ability to communicate efficiently with patients, using written assessment would likely not be valid for this; it would be like using a thermometer to measure blood pressure of a person.

The level of assessment is primarily determined by the intention of assessment or the construct that is being assessed. If the intention is to assess knowledge recall ('knows' level) or application of knowledge ('knows how' level) written assessments suit very well. However, written assessments are not the most suitable to assess hands-on skills. For hands-on or psychomotor skills, assessment requiring an assessor to observe the candidate is necessary, e.g. clinical or practical assessment as opposed to written assessment. If the observation is the candidate's behaviour in a simulated situation, then the level in the Miller's pyramid corresponds to 'shows how' level. Conversely, if the intention is to assess the candidate in the actual work setting, the level in the Miller's pyramid would be 'does' level.

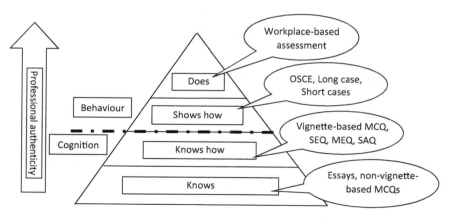

Fig. 1. Miller's pyramid for classification of assessment (After Miller GE, 1990).

It is apparent from the above description that Miller's pyramid has two levels for knowledge-related constructs and two levels for behaviour-related constructs. Why should there be two levels, instead of just one level for the knowledge-related constructs and one level for behaviour-related constructs? This is mainly to emphasise the importance of translation of learning into practice in health professions education. At the most basic level of cognition (i.e. 'knows' level), mainly factual knowledge is assessed. Although the possession of factual knowledge is an essential prerequisite for problem-solving, merely knowing that the candidate has the factual knowledge is not sufficient to conclude that they are able to translate knowledge into practice, e.g. solve problems in healthcare practice using the said factual knowledge. This makes any assessment programme that is confined to the 'knows' level severely constrained. Thus, assessment at the second level of cognition (i.e. 'knows how' level), where translating knowledge into practical situations is assessed, is another necessary part of an assessment programme. Similarly, at the first level of behaviour (i.e. 'shows how' level), the abilities are only assessed at a simulated level. It is only at the second level of behaviour (i.e. 'does' level) that the candidates are assessed in actual practice settings, i.e. real-life performance.

The next pertinent question would be why it is not possible to use only the two levels corresponding to the translated and real-life abilities (i.e. 'knows how' and 'does' levels) for the assessment. In fact, there is a good case for assessing mostly, if not solely, at the 'knows how' level. Many institutions now heavily favour assessment at 'knows how' level. There is an unwritten rule that even the most conservative of written assessments now strive to adhere to. That is the 20:80 rule: not more than 20% of written assessment should assess the 'knows' level and the rest of the assessment should assess at the 'knows how' level. However, the same cannot be said regarding the levels of behaviour, although one may rightly argue that what really matters is the assessment of 'does', rather than 'shows how'. This is especially so when a clear drop in ability has been shown when students move from 'shows how' level to 'does' level.[24] There are three issues that argue against such a move towards exclusive assessment at 'does' level. First, not all abilities can be assessed in actual practice settings for reasons of patient safety, e.g. cardiopulmonary resuscitation. Second, the assessment at this level (i.e. workplace-based assessment) is still not developed to a stage that the assessment at 'shows how' level can be safely overlooked. Third, and probably most importantly, when one seeks to provide feedback to the student about their performance to support and guide learning, the assessment at 'shows how' level (along with the 'knows' and 'knows how' levels) provides important information as to why certain strengths and weaknesses persist at the 'does' level.

Once the level of the Miller's pyramid is determined, then the most appropriate assessment tool has to be selected. This is similar to selecting the most appropriate type of sphygmomanometer to measure blood pressure of a given patient, once it is decided that sphygmomanometer is the most appropriate equipment. The decision on the exact instrument (e.g. the type of instrument — mercury, spring or electronic sphygmomanometer) is dependent on the key characteristics of the measurement that is required, e.g. how often the measurement should take place, who is measuring, in which position the measurement should be recorded, the physical size and age of the patient, etc. Similarly, when assessing at 'knows' level, single best answer-type multiple choice questions (MCQs) would be appropriate, especially if there is a large candidate cohort and a large content area to be covered. This type of assessment, however, is not suitable to assess the 'knows how' level (i.e. application of knowledge), if the said MCQs are not based on practice-based scenarios. Hence, to assess application of knowledge, context-rich (i.e. scenario-based single best answer) MCQs or extended matching items (EMIs) are the assessments of choice, especially if there is a large candidate cohort and an extensive curriculum to be assessed.[25] If a large candidate cohort has to be assessed on a vast content area, an assessment of choice at the 'shows how' level would be the Objective Structured Clinical Examination (OSCE). However, even few observed long cases with structured marking rubrics may be appropriate if there is sufficient examiner time to be spent per candidate and the intent is to assess a rather narrow content area (i.e. only a few disease conditions) in a small cohort of candidates. Finally, the 'does' level of Miller's pyramid offers a variety of assessment instruments such as mini-clinical evaluation exercise (mini-CEX), direct observation of procedural skills (DOPS), case-based discussions (CbD), multi-source feedback (MSF), etc. If the intention is to assess the candidate in the actual work setting, then any of the above instruments could be used, based on the type of ability under assessment. For example, if 'history taking ability' is to be assessed, mini-CEX would be the assessment of choice. Similarly, if the ability under assessment is procedural skills, DOPS would be the choice, whereas clinical reasoning could be better assessed with CbD and non-technical skills with MSF.

Once the level of the Miller's pyramid and the type of assessment instrument is selected, the next step is to develop (or construct) and deliver the assessment. This is similar to following the correct steps in the procedure protocol to measure blood pressure, e.g. right cuff size, correct application of the cuff over the artery selected to measure the pressure, right positioning of the patient, etc. There are excellent guides to developing almost all major assessment instruments such as MCQs[26] for 'knows' and 'knows how' levels and OSCEs[27] for 'shows how' level. However, the medical education literature is yet to come to terms concretely with the best practices of assessment at 'does' level, i.e. workplace-based assessment. Since the best practices of constructing assessment at other levels are well established, we wish to discuss, in this chapter, some of the pressing issues related to assessment at 'does' level, i.e. workplace-based assessment.

As the name suggests, workplace-based assessment is a form of assessment that assesses the candidate in their workplace, by persons (i.e. examiners) who come into contact with the candidates in their day-to-day business. Such persons or examiners range from supervisors, other healthcare workers, senior colleagues, peers and patients. Basically, the candidate collects ratings and qualitative comments or feedback from the above assessors over the course of their training period, during their daily professional activities. The most commonly used assessment forms are:

1. Mini-CEX — the candidate is assessed by a supervisor during a 10 to 20-minute encounter with a patient using a structured rating form. Basic abilities assessed are history taking, physical examination, clinical reasoning and the associated non-technical abilities, e.g. communication skills, professionalism, organisational skills.[28]

2. DOPS or Procedure-based Assessment (PBA) — the candidate is assessed by a supervisor during a 15–25-minute patient encounter using a structured rating form. The abilities assessed are procedural skills and the associated non-technical abilities.[29]

3. CbD or Chart Stimulated Recall (CSR) — the candidate is assessed in a 15 to 20-minute encounter with a supervisor, based on a record of a patient who has been clerked and/or managed by the candidate. The main ability assessed here are the clinical reasoning skills.[30]

4. MSF or 360-degree Assessment[29] — the candidate is assessed using a structured rating form by a variety of health professionals (other than the supervisors), with whom the candidate has worked with, e.g. nurses and other healthcare professionals, colleagues, peers. The main abilities assessed comprise non-technical abilities such as teamwork, attitudes, communication skills and professionalism.

5. Patient surveys — the candidate is assessed by patients with whom the candidate has interacted, using a structured form to assess the non-technical abilities (e.g. empathy, ethics, communication skills, professionalism, etc.) of the candidate.[31]

There are a few points to be noted about the above list of workplace-based assessments. First, the above list is not exhaustive. Rather, they are the commonest used workplace-based assessments. Second, the first three assessments on this list are distinctly different from the last two.

- The first three assessments involve the supervisor of the candidate, as opposed to a non-supervisor in the latter two.

- The first three assessments produce a single structured rating form during each candidate–examiner encounter. However, the latter two assessments produce one rating form per assessor, based on one or several encounters (usually several, except possibly patient surveys) with the candidates. Thus, the first three (i.e. single encounter) assessments involve direct observation of the candidate performance, but the latter two (i.e. usually multiple encounters) assessments involve recall of the previous observations of candidate performance.
- Each encounter in the first three is followed by a feedback session with the examiner/supervisor. In the latter two, usually, there are no such feedback sessions with the raters/examiners. Feedback based on the latter two would only take place when the candidate's overall progression is discussed with the supervisor.
- The first three assessments assess both non-technical and technical abilities, whereas the latter two assessments only assess the non-technical abilities.

Third, although they are commonly called rating forms, all these forms also include space for qualitative comments about the candidate ability. Fourth, one of the most important principles behind workplace-based assessment is that any 'one' workplace-based assessment encounter is not used on its own to decide on the ability of the candidate. Rather, information from all the assessment forms (and where permitting all the types of forms) should be collated before any decision about the candidate ability is made. However, individual assessment forms should be used for feedback purposes.

B. How Should the Workplace-based Assessment Be Constructed and Delivered?

Following is a discussion on some of the key considerations that should be deliberated and decided upon before implementing any type of workplace-based assessment.

Number of encounters or assessment forms

The number of rating forms needed to produce a defensible estimate of the candidate ability differs widely from one type of workplace-based assessment to another. In any of the workplace-based assessments, each assessment form is completed by a single assessor, and hence the number of assessment forms would mean the number of assessors.

The literature generally suggests that for mini-CEX, minimally four[32] to five[33] assessors; for DOPS, three assessors[32]; and for CbD, around 10 assessors[34] be sufficient to achieve acceptable reliability. However, for MSF, the number of assessors required would depend on the type of assessor. The number could be as low as five nurses or 23 medical students.[35] That said, in general, the number of assessors for many MSF assessments would be in the range of 11–13.[31,32,36,37] For patient surveys, although the Joint Royal College of Physicians Training Board[38] suggests 20 patients, studies have shown that the number could be as high as 36[31] or even 41.[37]

This variation in the number of assessors required to achieve acceptable reliability can be explained by the factors inherent in a given workplace-based assessment. Assessments such as mini-CEX, DOPS or CbD are based on a collection of single, directly observed encounters, assessing predominantly technical skills, mostly conducted by assessors with some training to assess such skills. These technical assessments require a comparatively lower number of assessors to achieve acceptable reliability. Conversely, assessments based on recall of information from multiple previous observations, such as MSF and patient surveys, assessing predominantly non-technical skills, by assessors who may not always be trained in assessing such skills, require comparatively a larger number of assessors. It is fair to state that 'diagnosing' competence is a cognitive activity similar to diagnosing a disease condition of a patient. A clinician with a higher level of expertise may require a lesser amount of information than a novice to arrive at the same diagnosis. Also, it has been found that a change in the rubric criteria from more educational jargon ('highly proficient') to more practice-related jargon — for example, by asking where the supervisor would want to be if the candidate performed a certain activity (i.e. in the same room ready to intervene, on-site but not in the same room, in the hospital, at home) — has a considerable effect on the number of observations needed to achieve a reliable outcome.[39] Finally, it should be stressed that all the above figures are context-dependent.[40,41] Hence, any implementer of workplace-based assessment should take the above numbers of assessors only as a general guideline. This means that the implementers should carry out their own reliability studies to find out the optimum number of assessors per each assessment instrument.

The structure of the rating rubrics

Almost all workplace-based assessments use Likert-type rating scales to rate candidates on different aspects of candidate behaviour observed by the assessor. The ideal number of rating points (or categories) on such a rating scale is not a new debate. Psychometrically speaking, the more the rating points, the higher the reliability,[42] given all other confounders (e.g. examiner ability, complexity of task, etc.) are optimal. However, a rating scale needs to be manageable for the examiner, i.e. the examiners should be able to tell apart two adjacent rating points or rating categories. If not, the variance introduced by the higher number of rating points would be mainly based on rating error. In general, it is considered that a person can manipulate 7 ± 2 categories in their working memory.[43] Hence, increasing the number of rating points excessively (e.g. beyond 9 points) may be counterproductive.[44] For example, having 100 rating points on a rating scale is the same as requesting the examiners to provide a percentage score for the candidate ability. As such, the most popular scales have 4–5 rating points or categories. Favouring a lower number of rating points (e.g. 5 instead of 9) makes sense for at least three reasons. First, recent literature indicates that the number of categories that a person could handle in the working memory is even lower than the previously accepted 7 ± 2.[45] Second, the examiners who rate the candidates while engaging in their day-to-day work cannot be expected to handle an excessively large number of rating points. Third, increasing the rating points excessively would make it extremely difficult to write the necessary descriptors to anchor all the rating points.

For an accurate differentiation of two adjacent rating points, not only does the number of rating points need to be manageable, but also each rating point should be labelled (e.g. 0 = very poor; 1 = poor; 2 = average; 3 = good; 4 = excellent). Additionally, each label should preferably be anchored by a descriptor that describes the typical candidate behaviour. As stated before, there is evidence to suggest that when such candidate behaviour is written as a narrative that the examiners can readily relate to (e.g. I can leave the operating room when the trainee operates, trainee needs to be assisted and directly supervised when he/she operates), rather than focusing on abstract parts of the behaviour (e.g. completed most of the steps of the procedure) or negative behaviour (e.g. did not perform the procedure fluently and smoothly), the examiner judgements tend to be more valid and reliable.[46–48]

The general guideline is to label all rating points and anchor each of them with an appropriate descriptor. However, there are exceptions to this, such as the global rating scales. A global rating scale is used to assess the overall ability of the candidate, based on all the behaviours observed. In such an instance, for some global rating scales including labels and/or descriptors may not be feasible or may not work at all. Also, there are some instances where not every rating point, but only every other or every third rating point, is anchored by a label and/or a descriptor. This is especially the case if there are no valid descriptors for certain rating points, due to the complexity or the nature of the task being rated. There is no right or wrong answer to any of the above practices; it all depends on the situation. It is essential, however, that those who develop and/or use a particular type of rating scale should be able to justify their practice.

The next consideration would be whether the rating points should constitute an odd number or an even number. The general guideline for this decision is the consideration whether the examiners should be allowed to stay undecided about the candidate ability or not. Such a non-decision usually corresponds to the mid-point of an odd-number scale. For example, consider a 5-point rating scale, where 0 = very poor; 1 = poor; 2 = average; 3 = good; 4 = excellent. Here, the rating point 2 indicates an ability level that is neither acceptable nor unacceptable. In contrast, an even-number scale generally does not offer the examiners the option for remaining neutral or non-committal. However, that is if the rating scale is designed symmetrically. If the rating scale is designed non-symmetrically (i.e. an equal number of rating points is not available on either side of the rating that denotes a non-committal decision about the candidate ability), then even the rating scales with an even number of rating points could also provide the option for the examiners to be non-committal on the candidate ability, provided there is a rating point for the said non-committal decision. For example, consider the following 4-point rating scale: 0 = poor; 1 = average; 2 = good; 3 = excellent. Here, rating 1 denotes a non-committal decision.

So, the decision on the number of rating points is strongly related to the scale being balanced or unbalanced, i.e. symmetrical or non-symmetrical. When it is known that most candidates demonstrate acceptable performance or most assessors tend to award higher ratings (i.e. 'doves' as opposed to 'hawks' then the assessment designers may resort to an unbalanced scale, where the rating points (or categories) that describe acceptable performance would be more than those that describe unacceptable performance. This is done in an effort to differentiate the candidates who have higher and lower levels of performance among those that have been awarded ratings of acceptable performance. The 4-point rating scale described in the previous paragraph is an example of such a rating scale. Similarly, the number of rating points on the unacceptable side of the scale could also be increased for the opposite reasons described above, e.g. most candidates are known to display poor performance or most examiners are too strict.

Use of rating scales and examiner training

Any rating scale, however well-developed it may be, is only as good as how well it is used. This means that the assessors should be truly familiar with the purposes and functions of workplace-based assessment and the rating scale it entails. Unlike standardised assessment, training (i.e. calibrating) the assessors to score the same candidate performance similarly is not the main aim in workplace-based assessment for three reasons. First, one of the primary characteristics of any workplace is the unpredictability of the patient mix that one may encounter each day. Hence, the workplace cannot be standardised, and the workplace-based assessment has to capture this unique unstandardised nature of the workplace. Thus, training the assessors to assess an unknown combination of patients would be not practical.

Second, the number of assessors who would take part in workplace-based assessment would be innumerable, ranging from patients through other healthcare professionals to supervisors. If so, it is practically impossible to train all the assessors for all possible patient encounters. Third, even if it is possible to train all assessors, overly training or calibrating the assessors would be an attempt to artificially control the natural variation of assessor standards. This does not argue well, as one of the strengths of workplace-based assessment is its ability to represent varying viewpoints of different raters or assessors. If, however, the assessors could be adequately sampled, a well-represented and reliable measure of the candidate ability could be obtained, without resorting to excessive examiner training and standardisation of workplace-based assessment encounters.

That being said, at least in rating scales that involve supervisors as assessors, it would be good if the assessors are informed as to how best a rating scale should be scored. This is because these supervisor-led assessments, unlike the other workplace-based assessments that mostly seek the assessor perceptions, are mainly concerned with technical abilities that have 'industry-standards', which are agreed upon by professional bodies, e.g. what is a good history of a patient with myocardial infarction, how to examine the abdomen, etc. Hence, it is reasonable to expect sufficient agreement among the assessor community as to what a good performance should be. For this purpose, discussing rating scale descriptors and agreeing upon their meaning is an essential minimum required from an assessor of technical abilities. Additionally, it is also good if the assessing supervisors are aware of some of the rater biases that are well documented in the literature. The following is a brief description some of these well-known rater biases.[49]

1. Halo/Horns effect — masking of the actual candidate ability by an unwanted candidate characteristic (e.g. way of speech, dress, etc.), which may bring about either a positive (halo) or a negative (horns) result.
2. Central tendency — the inclination of the assessors to score candidates in a non-committal manner, by unjustifiably selecting the neutral or undecided rating point for most candidates, and/or by unjustifiably averting the extreme rating points (e.g. excellent and very poor).
3. Leniency error — the natural tendency of certain assessors to score candidates higher than their true ability and/or the tendency of certain assessors to avoid awarding failing grades.
4. Stringency error — the natural tendency of certain assessors to score candidates lower than their true ability and/or the tendency to avoid awarding higher rating points.

5. Contrast error — when scoring a mediocre candidate after scoring a series of poor or very poor candidates, the tendency of the assessor to rate the mediocre candidate higher than his/her true ability. The same error may occur in the opposite direction when a mediocre candidate is encountered after a series of good or excellent candidates. Sometimes examiners also tend to contrast candidate performance with their own performance.

6. Logical error — when certain competencies are related to each other by their very nature (e.g. communication skills and professionalism), the assessors may score a competency higher (or lower) than that the candidate deserves, due to the candidate's superior (or inferior) performance in another related competency.

7. Proximity effect — when two distinct abilities or competencies are rated one after the other in quick succession, performance of the former behaviour may affect the score of the other that is performed subsequently. This is also known as the 'recency effect'.

8. Primacy effect — when the first impressions or the rating that was awarded first in an encounter biases the subsequent decisions/ratings.

Hence, some training and calibration of assessors using video-based, simulated or hypothetical patient scenarios would be very useful.

Translating the candidate performance into a rating

Even for a well-trained experienced assessor using a well-constructed rating scale, workplace offers special challenges. These challenges are related to the naturalistic nature of workplace-based assessment. Given the diversity of patient encounters and the diversity in the levels of training of different candidates, how should an assessor score a candidate? When scoring a candidate, the assessor's thought process should basically be guided by the following two considerations:

1. Difficulty of the encounter
2. Standard that the candidate needs to achieve

The first consideration can be facilitated by offering the examiners a common understanding on the type of encounters that must be considered 'difficult', 'moderately difficult' and 'easy'. Therefore, examiner training (or at least an examiner guideline providing examples of 'difficult', 'moderate' and 'easy' cases) is crucial in this regard. If such examiner training is not offered, it is likely that a large number of ratings from a large number of examiners (i.e. large number of encounters) will have to be collected to generate reliable scores. Collection of such large numbers is not only impractical but resource intensive. Using examiner guidelines and investing in examiner training may hence be more efficient.

The second consideration is not as difficult as the first consideration if the examination authority clearly communicates the expected standard to all examiners and candidates. Here again, there are two options:

2a. The standard expected from each encounter is the final standard (i.e. level of competency at graduation) required from a graduating candidate, irrespective of the stage of training of the candidate, i.e. the standard is related to the exit standard.

2b. The standard expected from each encounter is the standard expected at the candidate's stage of training, i.e. the standard is related to level of training of the candidate.

In the case of 2a, if it is postgraduate education, for example, then the standard should be that of a day-one specialist. In this case, however, the candidates should be warned that their scores in the initial years could be low. This is because the candidates are not expected to achieve the maximum score (i.e. denoting the expected level of ability at the end of training) during the initial stages of their training. If, however, the examiners decide to score candidates taking into account the stage of training (i.e. option 2b above), then, the candidates could achieve maximum scores even in the first year. This is because the expected maximum level of ability is that expected from a trainee at that stage of their training.

Although there is little empirical evidence as to which method of interpreting a workplace-based assessment scale is better, there are many good reasons in favour of 2a, as opposed to 2b. The following are the most obvious of these reasons:

- Since the same examiner will have to assess candidates at different stages of training, it will be next to impossible to carry in the examiner heads (i.e. remember) the expected standard for each stage of training. It will be far easier to commit to memory just one final standard and judge each candidate against this final standard.

- One of the main sources of error in workplace-based assessment is associated with the need to adapt to the difficulty of individual cases when judging a candidate's performance. Moreover, if the examiners are also required to modulate their scores based on the stage of training of the candidate, juggling these two variables (i.e. case difficulty and candidate's stage of training) concurrently can become too complicated to be carried out during everyday practice. Hence, the best solution would be to fix one of the variables. Since the case difficulty cannot be fixed in the workplace setting, a workable solution would be to fix the standard against which the ratings are awarded.

When fixing the standard expected, the only logical option would be to fix it at the expected level by the end of training.

- Follow up on the progress of candidates will be easier with a single standard. For example, the trajectory or the slope of the graph that plots the candidate scores over time could be simply interpreted visually if all scores are relative to a single final standard.

- Crossley and Jolly[50] in their recommendations for improving the validity and reliability of workplace-based assessment also support a notion similar to 2a. They recommend that the assessment should assess the quality of performance rather than the suitability of the trainee for a particular stage of training. More importantly, a decision on the candidate ability based on the expected final standard would dissociate the ability of the candidate for the duration of training. This is a fundamental requirement of true competency-based education, as opposed to time-based education.

Formative versus summative assessment

Conventionally, the literature recommends the implementation of workplace-based assessment as formative assessment.[33] This is mainly due to the key role that feedback and continuous improvement play in workplace-based assessment. For feedback to work well, there should be a sufficiently non-threatening, relaxed (i.e. stress-free) environment. If the candidates' thought process is preoccupied with the desire to score high, then they may not be in a mood to expose their weaknesses during the assessment and engage in an open discussion with the assessor. A second important consideration supporting the adoption of workplace-based assessment as formative assessment is the fact that more often than not, the assessor is also the supervisor of the candidate. So, there is potential for conflict of interest when one person assumes these disparate roles of supervisor and assessor in quick succession, especially if the de-rolling of one before assuming the other is inadequate or impractical. The third consideration is the varying assessment material and varying assessors. Though this variation in assessment material and assessors in itself should not be an issue if there is adequate sampling of workplace-based assessment encounters, often the resources preclude the implementation of such an elaborate workplace-based assessment system that includes a sufficient number of encounters with varying assessment material and assessors. Hence, in such situations, the variation of assessment material and assessors is also an issue disfavouring the use of workplace-based assessment for summative purposes.

Although all the above reasons argue against the use of workplace-based assessment for summative purposes, there is one consideration that strongly influences many assessment systems to consider workplace-based assessment as summative assessment, at least to a degree. This consideration is basically the 'assessment drives learning' effect. Often, the reason given by many authorities for implementing workplace-based assessment as summative assessment is that it is only then that both the candidates and assessors take this type of assessment seriously. Hence, some assessment systems in medical education attempt to introduce a summative element to the predominantly formative workplace-based assessment. Such introductions range from formally assigning a substantial weightage to the workplace-based assessment scores in the summative assessment system to making the completion of workplace-based assessment (to a desired level, as stipulated by the examination committee) a prerequisite to sit the summative assessment.

There is no evidence to suggest the best practice in this formative–summative dilemma. The considerations raised above are mostly contextual. That is, for example, if the assessment culture in a particular setting is mostly competitive and score-driven, then the candidates will not take an entirely formative workplace-based assessment seriously. Hence, it is best that the examination committees and implementers take the most appropriate option, specific to their context, by weighing the pros and cons of the different options discussed above. It should also be stressed that this formative–summative dichotomy turns far less important in the face of programmatic assessment.[51]

C. How Should the Workplace-based Assessment Results Be Interpreted?

The interpretation of workplace-based assessment results is primarily dependent on whether the results are considered for formative or summative purposes.

First, if the workplace-based assessment is purely for formative purposes, comparing the candidate scores on similar cases, collected over a period of time would be the best, to identify whether the candidate has been improving their performance over time. For this, plotting all assessment encounter scores on a graph, where the x-axis is time at which assessment has taken place and the y-axis is the candidate scores for each encounter, would prove useful to identify the trajectory of improvement. Any plateauing or decline of the graph should be then investigated further to find out the reasons for such a performance drop. This would provide valuable information for both the candidates and the trainers to initiate remedial action.

Second, if there is a summative element in workplace-based assessment, then interpretation of workplace-based assessment results essentially boils down to a standard setting process. However, unlike standard setting of traditional assessment where the assessment material is a constant, workplace-based assessment involves varying assessment material. Hence, one has to assume that the workplace-based assessment material would comprise a sufficient number of encounters capturing the entire range of difficulty levels and case variations, so that the difficulty level of all material would, on average, be similar from candidate to candidate. Thus, there is a necessity to sample widely in workplace-based assessment. Given the above assumption, there are several options available for the examination boards to decide how much of a score is adequate:

1. Consensually deciding which candidates have made the mark (i.e. passed or achieved the expected standard) by considering all the individual workplace-based assessment scores by a team of examiners.

2. Deciding based on the overall score of all workplace-based assessments of a candidate and using a measure of central tendency (e.g. mean, median) of all workplace-based assessment scores.

3. Calculating competency scores for each candidate, based on a pre-agreed formula.

Following is a brief discussion on the pros and cons of the above options:

1. *Consensual decision on the candidate ability by perusing the individual ratings*

The strength of this option is that the examination board or committee can consider all assessment scores and give due consideration to the different stages of training, during which these scores have been achieved. For example, an examination board would assign a lower weight to a candidate scoring poorly during their early training, as long as their end-of-training scores are above the expected level of ability. Usually, the rating scales will provide the labels and descriptors for each rating to indicate whether a given rating is above or below the expected level of ability. Also, the examination board can consider the qualitative comments of the examiners to decide the difficulty level of an encounter before interpreting whether a particular rating is poor or difficult. This type of decision-making can be considerably aided by scrutinising the graphs, described previously, that profile the candidate ability over time.

However, the downside of this type of decision-making is the provision of too wide decision-making powers to the examination boards without reasonable benchmarks and guidelines to rely on. If such decision-making is not guided/moderated by proper guidelines and benchmarks, the decision-making process could either produce unjustifiably variable results at best or be perceived as open for misuse at worst. This will be a substantial threat not only to face validity, but also to consequential validity.[20] Ideally, such guidelines should indicate the minimally acceptable workplace-based assessment profiles of a safe candidate, with a clear rationale as to how these minimum standards have been decided upon. For example, how many encounters a candidate is expected to score above the expected level of ability during the later stages of training, what should be the definition of the later stages of training, etc.? Also, when deciding based on such an open-consensus generation process, the importance of proper documentation of each consideration and each step of the process that contributes to a decision cannot be overemphasised.

2. *Decision based on an overall central tendency score*

This method simply calculates the mean or the median of all the assessment scores that a candidate has received throughout the training at a given workplace-based assessment. This is the simplest and most straightforward, as it removes to a greater extent the prerogative or the decision-making power from the examination authority such as an examination board. Hence, at least any perceived conflicts of interest are reduced to a minimum. The implicit assumption in the adoption of this option is that over many encounters, the passing candidate's average/median score based on all encounters should be more than the rating for 'meets expectation' (or a similar label/descriptor denoting the minimum acceptable level of ability) of the rating scale used for a given workplace-based assessment. The rationale of this is contingent upon another assumption that all candidates would have encountered an equal proportion of similar conditions; e.g. an equal proportion of lenient and stringent examiners. In that case, each candidate has to be scored on a sufficiently high number of encounters before any decision making is attempted.

However, this option has its own shortcomings. The commonest central tendency measure is the mean. The mean is notorious to be unduly affected by extreme values. So, just one encounter that a candidate performs poorly will unduly diminish the candidate's mean and hence the overall ability score. The reverse possibility is equally true; i.e. one excellent performance pushing the mean towards an acceptable level of ability. Median in this sense is a better measure, but this will lack information on the extent to which the scores of other encounters varied from the median. So, if a measure of central tendency is used to decide the ability of a candidate, then such a measure should be interpreted along with a suitable measure of dispersion; e.g. standard deviation or range. This apart, some of the issues that were outlined previously in option 1 also hold for this option. For example, if all encounters are considered for the calculation of the central tendency measure, then the lower ratings in the initial stages of training will reduce the overall score. So, the acceptable score on the rating scale (e.g. rating point 2 on a 0–4 rating scale, where 2 denotes 'meets expectation') would no longer be applicable when interpreting the overall score. Hence, a suitable norm for the acceptable standard should be adopted after analysing the scores of several cohorts of candidates at different stages of training. If, however, such analysis to find a normalised standard is too cumbersome, then the examination board could use the scores from only the later stages of training. Then again, a clear definition of 'later stages of training' should be agreed upon. Also, such reduction of encounters may not provide a sufficient number of encounters to generate a stable measure of central tendency.

There is very little evidence available to suggest the best way to use the measures of central tendency when interpreting workplace-based assessment results. In one study, Boerebach et al.,[52] after comparing four different measures (including the mean and the median) from 10 ratings per year of two candidates for 2 years, concluded that the proportion of substandard performances (or ratings) provided the best discriminatory measure. However, all ratings of both candidates achieved satisfactory ratings in the later half of the year in both years. So, in this sense, the discriminatory effect was mostly based on the initial ratings of each year. Such evidence should contribute to the debate whether initial ratings should actually be considered for any decision making or should be entirely left for formative purposes.

3. *Decision based on competency scores*

This option involves some post-assessment work in partialling-out scores of workplace-based encounters of a given candidate to different competencies. Such partialling should be carried out based on an agreed framework for allocating the sub-scores or itemised ratings achieved by different items (or behaviours/abilities or competencies) within an encounter. For example, if a mini-CEX total score comprises several itemised ratings on medical interviewing (i.e. history taking) skills, communication skills, professionalism, etc., then the itemised ratings (i.e. competency scores) for each competency from all encounters of a given candidate should be tabulated in a table such as Table 3. The total score for each competency, based on different

Table 3. Calculation of competency scores using workplace-based assessment ratings.

Mini-CEX encounters	Competencies (i.e. ratings) within an encounter				
	History taking	Communication	Professionalism	...	Overall/ Global
Mini-CEX 1					
Mini-CEX 2					
Mini-CEX 3					
Mini-CEX 4					
Total competency score					

encounters, is then calculated by adding all ratings within each column. These column totals are the competency scores of a given candidate.

Similar tables for the same candidate should be created for other workplace-based assessments; e.g. DOPS. Where possible (i.e. where similar competencies have been assessed in different workplace-based assessments), the competency scores of different workplace-based assessments should be then combined (e.g. averaged or totalled) to compute the grand competency scores; e.g. the combined score for communication skills based on all encounters of mini-CEX, DOPS and MSF. These scores will provide the examination board with a bird's eye view of the overall performance of the candidate. The expected minimum score for each competency can also be prefixed (i.e. standard set) by the examination board, so that it is clear to all stakeholders the level that the candidate should achieve.

Although the above options are described as three separate approaches, in practice, any decision-maker could use all three options to justify a decision. In fact, such a decision-making process that involves triangulation of information from different sources, measures and data analysis approaches would perhaps be the most defensible option available to a decision-maker such as an examination board. Nonetheless, all these options will not be able to circumvent adequately the key issue that haunts all decisions made based on workplace-based assessments. That is, as discussed under the second option above (i.e. 'decision based on an overall central tendency score'), the non-availability of a validated method to collate workplace-based ratings derived from different stages of learning. Leaving such collation and interpretation of the collated data entirely in the hands of few examination committee or examination board members, without any clear guideline to follow, will seriously challenge the defensibility of the assessment decision. This would be so, even if workplace-based assessments had contributed little to the overall assessment decision, which eventually would have considered other end-of-training assessments such as OSCEs, MCQs, etc.

So, the take-home message of the above discussion is that there should be clear guidelines to collate and interpret the workplace-based assessments before they are used to make any decision on the candidate overall ability. We are not aware of such guidelines in the literature. Hence, developing such guidelines, though not easy, would be the need of the hour.

Out of the three options discussed here for interpreting workplace-based assessment results, the latter two options are mainly focused on interpreting scores within a quantitative framework, whereas the first option operates more within a qualitative framework. However, even decisions mostly based on qualitative methods would need sound and defensible guidelines. Decisions based on qualitative methods without proper guidelines would be akin to conducting qualitative research without following the rules of coding and synthesising codes into themes. Even if such rules (or guidelines) for collation of workplace-based assessment results are developed in future, one needs to bear in mind that this process may have to be repeated for hundreds of candidates. This is as opposed to the handful of subjects on which qualitative research is conducted. So, if a qualitative basis is adopted for interpreting workplace-based assessments from all stages of training, then such a process is best reserved only for the borderline candidates with ambivalent results. This is assuming that the number of borderline candidates would be manageable. Even if that is the case, a technique such as a colour coding system within a suitable matrix to indicate the different ratings at different stages of training will aid the decision makers to visualise the total candidate performance both vividly and succinctly.

Finally, it needs to be stressed that even if the scores are used for summative decisions, still there should always be a formative element in every workplace-based assessment. This means even if the scores of workplace-based assessments are used to take summative decisions, feedback to the candidate after every workplace assessment encounter should be an integral part of the assessment process. There is also the possibility of viewing the summative and formative components in workplace-based assessment from a diametrically opposite perspective. That is workplace-based assessment with feedback could be considered most useful if the summative part of the assessment constitutes the extent to which the feedback has been taken up and translated into learning goals and learning activities, whereas the formative part constitutes mainly the score or the rating. The latter is used, in this case, mainly to determine the trajectory of learning; i.e. improvement or otherwise. This is basically a call for considering the qualitative component of workplace-based assessment predominantly for summative purposes and the quantitative component predominantly for formative purposes.

D. Summary

As the operational guidelines for the assessment at the lower levels of Miller's pyramid are well established, this chapter concentrated on discussing some of the core issues in operationalising assessment at the topmost level of the pyramid; i.e. workplace-based assessment. Workplace-based assessment comprises a group of assessments that assess the candidates in their day-to-day work settings by a variety of assessors, ranging from supervisors to patients, that the candidates come into contact with, in their professional life. Feedback and continuous improvement of candidate ability should be the cornerstones of a sound workplace-based assessment system. When planning this type of assessment, one needs to plan for collecting an adequate number of assessments to capture the variability in the assessment material (i.e. caseload) and the assessors in the workplace, so that valid and reliable decisions on the candidate's ability could be made. Since the assessments are carried out mainly on a rating scale, the development of a proper rating rubric and communicating the same to both the candidates and the examiners are of paramount importance. When developing the rating rubrics, the key considerations should be deciding on the number rating points, the labelling of rating points and suitably anchoring the rating points using narrative descriptors that the examiners can readily relate to. Some examiner training, especially for the assessments that predominantly involve technical abilities, will be useful. When interpreting the rating scale for scoring candidates, considering the end-of-training ability as the expected level of ability, irrespective of the stage of training of the candidate, would help at least in two ways. Such a consideration would be helpful to: 1 simplify the assessment process for the assessors by providing them with a single benchmark to rate all candidates irrespective of their stage of training; and 2 offer an easily interpretable system to profile and track the candidate ability over time. Although workplace-based assessment was primarily developed for formative purposes, at least some have found that incorporating a summative element makes it more recognisable and meaningful. This is despite the drawbacks of considering these assessments for summative purposes. However, with the advent of programmatic assessment, the distinction between summative and formative assessment should be a lesser consideration. When collating and interpreting the workplace-based assessment scores to decide on the candidate's ability, it is absolutely important not to consider any individual assessment score or rating in a standalone manner to make any decision. Instead, all assessment scores should be considered when taking decisions on the candidate ability. Out of the many options available for such a decision-making process, perhaps a more defensible option would be to base the decisions on competency scores from all assessment instruments, where possible. However, the best option, resources permitting, is to triangulate multiple data analysis approaches. The main barrier to effective decision-making in workplace-based assessment is the lack of a robust method to collate and interpret candidate scores drawn from different stages of training rather than the same (or the final) stage of training. Whether such collation and interpretation of workplace-based assessment data are carried out using quantitative, qualitative or mixed methods, clear guidelines for the decision-makers are a must.

Practice Highlights

- Drawing parallels between the principles of educational assessment and clinical practice helps clarify the underpinning rationale of assessment.
- Often in practice, an assessment has both formative and summative functions. This is not unacceptable, as long as the tensions between the formative and summative purposes are appropriately managed.

- When scoring candidates, the examiners should not consider whether the assessment is formative or summative. It is when interpreting the results that the formative or summative purposes of assessment need to be considered.

- When addressing content validity, using a blueprint, it is important not only to ensure the representativeness of all columns and rows (i.e. all learning outcomes and content areas) in the blueprint, but also to verify the relative representation within each column and each row.

- Whether collation and interpretation of workplace-based assessment data are carried out using quantitative, qualitative or mixed methods, clear guidelines for the decision-makers are a must.

References

1. Cronbach LJ, Meehl PE. Construct validity in psychological tests. *Psychological Bulletin*. 1955; 52(4):281.

2. Downing SM, Haladyna TM. Validity threats: Overcoming interference with proposed interpretations of assessment data. *Medical Education*. 2004;38(3):327–33.

3. Eva KW, Cunnington JP, Reiter HI, Keane DR, Norman GR. How can I know what I don't know? Poor self assessment in a well-defined domain. *Advances in Health Sciences Education: Theory and Practice*. 2004;9(3):211–24.

4. Guion RM. Content validity — The source of my discontent. *Applied Psychological Measurement*. 1977;1(1):1–10.

5. Hamdy H. Blueprinting for the assessment of health care professionals. *The Clinical Teacher*. 2006;3(3):175–9.

6. Cronbach LJ, Shavelson RJ. My current thoughts on coefficient alpha and successor procedures. *Educational and Psychological Measurement*. 2004;64(3):391–418.

7. Norcini JJ, Shea JA. The credibility and comparability of standards. *Applied Measurement in Education*. 1997;10(1):39–59.

8. Cusimano MD. Standard setting in medical education. *Academic Medicine*. 1996;71(10):S112–20.

9. Schuwirth LW, Van der Vleuten CP. Programmatic assessment: From assessment of learning to assessment for learning. *Medical Teacher*. 2011;33(6):478–85.

10. Eva KW. On the generality of specificity. *Medical Education*. 2003;37(7):587–8.

11. Notar CE, Zuelke DC, Wilson JD, Yunker BD. The table of specifications: Insuring accountability in teacher made tests. *Journal of Instructional Psychology*. 2004;31(2):115–129.

12. Tengberg M. Validation of sub-constructs in reading comprehension tests using teachers' classification of cognitive targets. *Language Assessment Quarterly*. 2018;15(2):169–82.

13. Lynn MR. Determination and quantification of content validity. *Nursing Research*. 1986;35(6):382–6.

14. Kane MT. Current concerns in validity theory. *Journal of Educational Measurement*. 2001;38(4):319–42.

15. Association AER, Association AP, Education NCoMi, Educational JCoSf, Testing P. Standards for educational and psychological testing: American Educational Research Association; 1999.

16. Sireci SG. The construct of content validity. *Social Indicators Research*. 1998;45(1–3):83–117.

17. Messick S. Validity. In: Linn R, editor. *Educational Measurement*. New York: Macmillan Publishing; 1989:13–103.

18. Cronbach L. Test validation. In: Thorndike RL, editor. *Educational Measurement*. Washington, DC: American Council on Education; 1971.

19. Messick S. The standard problem: Meaning and values in measurement and evaluation. *American Psychologist*. 1975;30(10):955–66.

20. Kane M. Current concerns in validity theory. Paper presented at the 81st Annual Meeting of the American Educational Research Association (New Orleans, LA, April 24–28, 2000).

21. Kane M, editor. *Validating score interpretations and use: Messick lecture. Language Testing Research Colloquium*. Cambridge: SAGE; 2011.

22. Cronbach LJ. Validity on parole: How can we go straight. *New Directions for Testing and Measurement*. 1980;5(1):99–108.

23. Miller GE. The assessment of clinical skills/competence/performance. *Academic Medicine*. 1990;65(9):S63–7.

24. Rethans JJ, Norcini JJ, Baron-Maldonado M, Blackmore D, Jolly BC, LaDuca T, et al. The relationship between competence and performance: Implications for assessing practice performance. *Medical Education*. 2002;36(10):901–9.

25. Schuwirth LW, Verheggen M, Van der Vleuten C, Boshuizen H, Dinant G. Do short cases elicit different thinking processes than factual knowledge questions do? *Medical Education*. 2001;35(4):348–56.

26. Paniagua M, Swygert K. *Constructing Written Test Questions for the Basic and Clinical Sciences*. Philadelphia, PA: National Board of Medical Examiners; 2016.

27. Khan KZ, Gaunt K, Ramachandran S, Pushkar P. The objective structured clinical examination (OSCE):AMEE guide no. 81. part II: organisation & administration. *Medical Teacher*. 2013;35(9):e1447–e63.

28. Norcini JJ, Blank LL, Duffy FD, Fortna GS. The mini-CEX: A method for assessing clinical skills. *Annals of Internal Medicine*. 2003;138(6):476–81.

29. Wragg A, Wade W, Fuller G, Cowan G, Mills P. Assessing the performance of specialist registrars. *Clinical Medicine*. 2003;3(2):131–4.

30. Maatsch J, Huang R, Downing S, Barker D. Predictive validity of medical specialty examinations. Final report to NCHSR Grant No: HS02039-04. 1983.

31. Campbell JL, Richards SH, Dickens A, Greco M, Narayanan A, Brearley S. Assessing the professional performance of UK doctors: An evaluation of the utility of the General Medical Council patient and colleague questionnaires. *BMJ Quality & Safety*. 2008;17(3):187–93.

32. Wilkinson JR, Crossley JG, Wragg A, Mills P, Cowan G, Wade W. Implementing workplace-based assessment across the medical specialties in the United Kingdom. *Medical Education.* 2008;42(4):364–73.

33. Norcini J, Burch V. Workplace-based assessment as an educational tool: AMEE Guide No. 31. *Medical Teacher.* 2007;29(9):855–71.

34. Pelgrim EA, Kramer AW, Mokkink HG, van den Elsen L, Grol RP, van der Vleuten CP. In-training assessment using direct observation of single-patient encounters: A literature review. *Advances in Health Sciences Education: Theory and Practices.* 2011;16(1):131–42.

35. Massagli TL, Carline JD. Reliability of a 360-degree evaluation to assess resident competence. *American Journal of Physical Medicine & Rehabilitation.* 2007;86(10):845–52.

36. Ramsey PG, Carline JD, Blank LL, Wenrich MD. Feasibility of hospital-based use of peer ratings to evaluate the performances of practicing physicians. *Academic Medicine.* 1996;71(4):364–70.

37. Murphy DJ, Bruce DA, Mercer SW, Eva KW. The reliability of workplace-based assessment in postgraduate medical education and training: A national evaluation in general practice in the United Kingdom. *Advances in Health Sciences Education: Theory and Practice.* 2009;14(2):219–32.

38. Joint Royal College of Physicians Training Board JRCPTB. Workplace based assessment. 2012.

39. Weller JM, Misur M, Nicolson S, Morris J, Ure S, Crossley J, et al. Can I leave the theatre? A key to more reliable workplace-based assessment. *British Journal of Anaesthesia.* 2014;112(6):1083–91.

40. Govaerts MJ, Schuwirth LW, Van der Vleuten CP, Muijtjens AM. *Workplace-based assessment:* Effects of rater expertise. *Advances in Health Sciences Education: Theory and Practice.* 2011;16(2):151–65.

41. Govaerts MJ, Van de Wiel MW, Schuwirth LW, Van der Vleuten CP, Muijtjens AM. Workplace-based assessment: raters' performance theories and constructs. *Advances in Health Sciences Education: Theory and Practice.* 2013;18(3):375–96.

42. Churchill Jr GA, Peter JP. Research design effects on the reliability of rating scales: A meta-analysis. *Journal of Marketing Research.* 1984;21(4):360–75.

43. Miller GA. The magical number seven, plus or minus two: Some limits on our capacity for processing information. *Psychological Review.* 1956;63(2):81.

44. Cox III EP. The optimal number of response alternatives for a scale: A review. *Journal of Marketing Research.* 1980;17(4):407–22.

45. Cowan N. Visual and auditory working memory capacity. *Trends in Cognitive Sciences.* 1998; 2(3):77.

46. Rekman J, Gofton W, Dudek N, Gofton T, Hamstra SJ. Entrustability scales: Outlining their usefulness for competency-based clinical assessment. *Academic Medicine.* 2016;91(2):186–90.

47. Beard JD, Marriott J, Purdie H, Crossley J. Assessing the surgical skills of trainees in the operating theatre: a prospective observational study of the methodology. *Health Technology Assessment.* 2011;15(1):i–xxi, 1–162.

48. Regehr G, Bogo M, Regehr C, Power R. Can we build a better mousetrap? Improving the measures of practice performance in the field practicum. *Journal of Social Work Education.* 2007;43(2):327–44.

49. Lösel F SM. Assessor's bias. In: Fernández-Ballesteros R, editor. *Encyclopedia of Psychological Assessment.* 2003;1:99–101.

50. Crossley J, Jolly B. Making sense of work-based assessment: Ask the right questions, in the right way, about the right things, of the right people. *Medical Education.* 2012;46(1):28–37.

51. Van der Vleuten CP, Schuwirth LW. Assessing professional competence: From methods to programmes. *Medical Education.* 2005;39(3):309–17.

52. Boerebach BC, Arah OA, Heineman MJ, Lombarts KM. Embracing the complexity of valid assessments of clinicians' performance: A call for in-depth examination of methodological and statistical contexts that affect the measurement of change. *Academic Medicine.* 2016;91(2):215–20.

SUPPORTING LEARNERS 'WHY IS MY STUDENT SO DIFFICULT TO HANDLE?'

Marcus A. Henning and Tan Chay Hoon

Scenarios

Peter was a resident well-liked by his peers and the healthcare team. He had a very pleasant personality and was enthusiastic about learning. However, his content knowledge and time-management skills in the subject area were poor and at least two of the specialists whom he had worked with during his clerkship had highlighted these. This was noted in their formal evaluation of Peter. However, he was unaware of his shortcomings.

Tim was a third-year medical student and was always late in coming to class and submitting assignments. He tended to keep very quiet during class discussions. It was also noted that his grades had been falling over the past semester, although he had very good grades in his first and second years. The Module Coordinator was concerned and was meeting Tim to discuss his behaviour.

Jeanne was one of the top students and on the Dean's list every year. She tended to dominate discussions and had little tolerance towards the opinions of other students. She completed most of the tasks on her own even though these tasks were mostly team-based. She refused to accept the feedback from her peers and insisted she was the one who always gets things done. The academic mentor would be meeting with Jeanne to discuss this.

Introduction

In the following sections, we have written three chapters to address the idea of *Supporting Learners 'Why is my Student so Difficult to Handle?'* Chapter 1 focuses on *why* students may be difficult to handle. The attributions of difficulty are likely multi-layered and complex. Therefore, we have used Hirsch's[1] framework to meaningfully describe potential sources of difficulty that could be attributed to the student and other extraneous sources. According to this framework, some of the key student factors that need to be investigated include (1) emotional and motivational willingness for change, (2) level of academic preparation, (3) familiarity and expertise with study enhancement strategies, (4) style of learning and/or (5) cognitive capacity. These factors are useful indicative starting points for academic counsellors to explore regarding the problems faced by students and the impact this has on their learning. The three scenarios illustrated above provide us with real-life examples of students who could be analysed using this framework. As is often the case, the reasons as to *why* students are perceived as being difficult go beyond this framework; nevertheless, the framework provided us with a diagnostic system for investigating some of the likely reasons as to why a student presents as being difficult.

In Chapter 2, we start to investigate *what* are some of the tools that faculty staff, counsellors and academic advisors could employ to support learners having trouble. We begin by exploring some of the University tools, and their programmes and strategies that could be used to support these learners. We explore the potentiality of mentoring, coaching and supervision, feedback systems, reflection, academic and personal counselling and learning contracts. We then consider the responsibilities of the learner, by investigating their career trajectory and intrinsic interest, and their use of exercise and well-being strategies. Each of the scenarios (cited above) provided us with a means by which we could explore how these strategies can be applied. In Chapter 3, we scrutinise *how* wider implications are addressed in relation to student support and institutional responsibilities. More specifically, we focus on university guidelines, ethical and moral issues, and the notion of the psychological contract.

Therefore, this section starts with a diagnostic framework, then recommends potential interventions that could be applied to students in difficulty and finally recognises some of the wider issues that impact on the process of student support. We have not explicitly delved into attributions related to family, community, faculty and the institution, but do recognize these factors as also being crucial to the understanding as to why a student may be perceived as being difficult.

Chapter 1: Why?

If we are to question 'why' a student behaves in a difficult way, we are making an inference according to a set of rules, preferences or norms. Or are these students simply failing the assessments that we have set? If the question becomes 'Why is my Student so Difficult to

Handle?', the implication is that the student being observed or referred to has broken either explicit or implicit rules. These rules are defined by the observer or evaluator, who may have a specific frame of reference that has either personal, professional or institutional agency. In his book, Hirsch[1] developed a framework for diagnosing and addressing 'difficulty' concerns related to students not coping within the university system and/or their course of study.

According to this framework, it is important to collect information about students' academic and non-academic background before any diagnosis or intervention is considered. It is Hirsch's[1] view that an academic counsellor needs to assess how situational factors are affecting a student's motivation to learn and their readiness for academic study. Consequently, we have adapted Hirsch's framework and developed this five-factor model for diagnosing difficulty (as explained below) to address concerns we may have about student behaviour.

1. *Emotional and motivational willingness for change* is a crucial factor in the process of educational adaptation. This factor recognises the interplay between emotional regulation and motivation, and incorporates consideration of both intrapersonal and interpersonal factors. In their chapter, Marroquín and Tennen[2] identify the importance of inculcating coping systems and developing emotional regulation when responding to situational demands, especially those considered adversarial. Coping is a valuable cognitive and behavioural process used to manage external or internal demands that surface in the learning environment, although it does need to be willingly activated. In addition, emotional regulation is a useful construct to employ to monitor, evaluate and modify emotional responses with the intention to achieve prescribed goals. Both coping and emotional regulation will require developing a person's self-concept, self-efficacy, self-worth and self-determination.[3]

   Interpersonal factors are crucial especially given that the study in medicine is often conducted in teams. A team will likely have a defined task and goal and people are assigned roles (informal or formal) within teams with the intention of completing a task.[4] Effective teams have the advantage of tackling and successfully finishing complex tasks that would be difficult to complete alone.[5] Other interpersonal factors that may need to be considered when appraising emotional and motivational willingness to change are the influences of family, friends and the wider community.[6]

2. *Level of academic preparation* is focused on adequate prior educational experience before entry into higher education. In a professional degree, this includes the knowledge, skills and attitudes acquired prior to their current level of learning. The assumption is that students continuously learn and adapt, ideally preparing them for the next step in their academic or professional development.[7] Prior learning needs to include content knowledge as well as procedural knowledge. If their prior knowledge

does not scaffold the next stage of learning, then disconnections can occur making progression difficult. This requirement fits well with the first factor, especially in the case of contributing to team work and patient care.[8] Investigating, evaluating and understanding levels of knowledge, skill competency and attitudes are crucial to understanding student difficulty.

3. *Student familiarity and expertise with study enhancement strategies* extends the evaluation of emotional and motivational levels of preparedness and considers a strategic approach to studying. One key strategic process often cited in the literature pertains to the use of self-regulation. Self-regulation involves meta-cognition components, such as planning, monitoring and modifying skill behaviour.[9] It also aims to appraise and enhance areas linked to concentration, self-testing, study aids and time management.[10] Self-regulation pertains to the development of self-management and the ways students develop cognitive skills.[9] Self-regulated learning provides a powerful framework for medical education as it is goal focused, clearly supports behaviour involved in completing tasks, involves the employment of effective and efficient learning strategies, allows for adaptation and modification of strategies through reflection and aims to develop optimal performance outcomes.[11]

4. The *notion of learning styles* is a contentious area of educational theory especially within medical education.[12] The proponents of learning style theory propose that students can differ in terms of information processing, learning preferences and/or personal characteristics.[13] This approach tends to argue that students can optimise their learning by using a particular sensory approach, such as kinaesthetic, auditory or visual modes of learning.[14] A further view considers how students approach learning, such as whether students use surface, strategic or deep approaches to learning.[15] An additional approach that has gained credibility involves the use of a multidimensional approach to learning.[16] There is an assertion that 'learning styles' and their use are linked with academic achievement,[17] although there are some educationalists who have a critical view of the usefulness of learning styles when linked with academic performance.[12]

5. *Cognitive capacity* refers to the ability to learn new material and to integrate this new learning with existing knowledge. In Hirsch's[1] framework, the focus is on learning disability, attention-related problems and mental health issues. At first glance the idea of learning disability being a concern for medical students appears to be unjustified, nevertheless there is a growing argument that some medical students and, thus, doctors are likely to have a learning disability with one estimate being 3% of medical students in the United States.[18] Learning disabilities are often seen as being intrinsically

oriented and likely to have a connection with central nervous system dysfunction and, are therefore, closely associated with learning difficulty.[19]

The additional considerations related to cognitive capacity include cognitive load and threshold. Cognitive load is a factor that is likely to affect learning and experiences of cognitive overload, which is prevalent amongst medical students and doctors.[20] This theory suggests that students and health professionals have a finite capacity to process information effectively and thus if information load exceeds this capacity then further processing is impaired.[20] Cognitive threshold relates to the idea that to be functional doctors a certain threshold of learning needs to be attained, such as having a certain amount of scientific knowledge.[21] The threshold concept is a useful framework for understanding how students incrementally learn and how they overcome conceptual blocks when encountering unfamiliar and complex tasks.[22] Hence, students and physicians are often faced with thresholds they need to overcome in order to progress in their competency level.[23]

The adapted version of Hirsch's framework[1] is a useful when asking the question, 'Why is my student so difficult to handle?' We will now apply this framework to the three aforementioned scenarios.

The Case of Peter

Our concerns are:
   a) His content knowledge in the subject area and time-management skills were poor
   b) His issues with content knowledge and time-management skills were highlighted and he has received formal feedback about these
   c) Even so he was unaware of his shortcomings

His strengths are:
   a) He was a resident well-liked by his peers and the healthcare team
   b) He had a very pleasant personality and was enthusiastic about learning

'Why is Peter so Difficult to Handle?'

To understand Peter's case in more detail we will look at the evidence and suggest areas that need further discovery.
   1. *Emotional and motivational willingness to change* — We need to first examine Peter's academic and non-academic history. As a 'resident' we assume that he has already

progressed in a residency programme and has met certain graduate medical education requirements and has already attained a certain level of clinical competency.[24] Therefore, we can assume that he is prepared for the intense medical-learning study environment. However, it has been established that his level of knowledge is not at the expected standard and that his time-management skills are awry. The question is, 'Why is he unaware at the residency level and/or unwilling to accept his shortcomings?' To answer these questions we need to explore external factors, such as financial-, social- and health-related well-being.

One place to start with Peter is to ascertain whether or not he is experiencing undue stress or burnout due to financial strain, and/or problems associated with balancing work, leisure and study time. Concerns with quality of life and burnout are commonly cited in the medical literature,[25,26] and some of the life events that predispose medical students and residents to experience these are linked to sleep deprivation, pressure of assessments, the need for perfectionism and so forth.[27]

In addition, a well-known model used to describe the cultivation of self-awareness is the Johari window.[28] According to this model, feedback has several possible outcomes. The optimal scenario is when issues are known to self and others and hence the communication of the problem is identifiable and all parties are aware of the issues that need to be addressed. This outcome is not present in the case of Peter as others know of his problems but he is seemingly unaware. On the face of it, the evidence suggests that Peter is likely experiencing a 'blind spot' in which his supervisor knows what is going on but he does not. The other two options, whereby Peter knows but the supervisors don't, or neither know, are improbable. Alternatively, if Peter does know but is unwilling to accept the feedback then there is a block in the 'open arena'. The open arena may be a likely source of the problem with this case, given that he has been explicitly and formally given feedback about his shortcomings. One of the issues in the case of Peter is whether or not his understanding of the problem areas can be synthesized with those of the supervisor. In addition, it would be useful to know how the feedback was conducted and how a follow-up session was organised.

2. *Level of academic preparation* — This is less likely an issue given that he is a resident and has likely received adequate training to progress to this level. However, one issue that is worrying in this case is that his content knowledge in the subject area is poor. This suggests that even if he has passed his prior exams then he likely has gaps in his existing knowledge. This is problematic given that he needs to be contributing

constructively to his team and patient care, and if his gaps in knowledge adversely affect these two areas, he may well be a safety risk.

3. *Familiarity and expertise with using study enhancement strategies* — To become a resident, it is assumed that he has developed good self-regulation strategies to meet the academic and non-academic recruitment of resident status. Nonetheless, his problems with time management, which is a self-regulation skill, needs to be addressed. To further appraise his time-management issues requires a systematic assessment by a peer, self or expert. With three sources of feedback we can ascertain the specific focus of the problem. For example, a questionnaire that itemises aspects of time management could be used.[29] The components devised by White et al.[29] may provide us with more in-depth understanding of where the specific time-management issues are placed.

4. *Application of learning styles* — An area worth considering is whether he has been using surface, strategic or deep learning styles in his past learning experiences. If his philosophy was just to pass the exams then he may be using a surface style of learning (a 'C's get degrees' approach). Dolmans et al.[30] investigated the use of different approaches to learning in reference to its effect on problem-based learning. They suggested that students often differ in the way they approach their studies, with students focussing more on understanding (deep learning) and others more on recall or reproduction (surface learning). Those students who focused more on understanding tended to integrate and critique prior learning to new knowledge acquisition. Dolmans et al. also implicated that the approach to learning is not necessarily intrinsic to the student and may be derived from a particular teaching method, student perception of the learning environment and/or student preferences for learning.

5. *Cognitive capability* — Clearly Peter is unaware of his issues with content knowledge and time management, and his affability may be a strategy that he has used in the past to mask these shortcomings. Achievement and time management are undoubtedly correlated, with Broadbent and Poon[31] reporting that 'time management, effort regulation, critical thinking and metacognitive strategies leads to higher academic outcomes within both online and traditional higher education environments'. Therefore, the issue is whether the problems associated with knowledge acquisition or the willingness to learn new information may be related to a learning disability, attention-related problem or mental illness. It may also be related to cognitive overload or the inability to meet the required cognitive threshold for this level of clinical practice. These considerations need to be investigated.

The Case of Tim

Our concerns are:

a) He was always late in coming to class and submitting assignments

b) He tended to keep very quiet during class discussions

c) His grades had been falling over the past semester

His strengths are:

a) He had very good grades in his first and second years

b) His module coordinator was concerned and was meeting with Tim to discuss his behaviour

'Why is Tim so Difficult to Handle?'

1. *Emotional and motivational willingness for change* — The evidence does not clearly show that he is unwilling to change, although the downward trend suggests that he is experiencing problems with his study. The lateness and uncommunicative signs could be symptomatic of an underlying issue that has an impact on falling grades. Attribution theory[32] informs us that three factors could relate to 'why' this lateness and uncommunicative behaviour has manifested itself. First, the locus of control relates to whether this behaviour change is due to internal (anxious about his ability to be a doctor) or external (familial pressure) reasons. Second, concerns the idea of stability, whereby success or failure can be determined by ability (fixed entity) and/or effort (malleable entity). If Tim feels a sense of being stuck in a pattern that cannot be changed then the source of being stuck needs to be explored. Third, the notion of 'controllability' suggests that Tim may not feel he has any control over the situation and his willingness to change is no longer in his own hands.

2. *Level of academic preparation* — Given that he has achieved very good grades in his first and second years, it is unlikely that his academic preparation is impaired. Nevertheless, the course structure and the way material is being taught may have shifted in the third year of study. Genn[33] proposed that medical schools provide a habitat that can be described as 'big buzzing confusion, a complex, chaotic kind of situation, with countless components, myriad dynamics and interactions of inputs and processes, inevitable conflicts, and constantly in a state of flux'. The ever-changing learning landscape is likely to affect students differently, and if the change from years 1 and 2 to year 3 is a dramatic shift in content learning and teaching then this may be a source of 'why' this student may be struggling.

3. *Use of study enhancement strategies* — An academic advisor needs to ascertain the types of strategies he is using especially given his problems with lateness and inconsistent grade achievement. He could fill in a LASSI (Learning and Study Strategies Inventory) questionnaire, which can provide useful information regarding use of self-regulated strategies.[34]

4. *Application of learning styles* — This aspect of diagnosis is linked to the previous point of investigation. Billett[35] has articulated the issues associated with learning within the healthcare workplace environment. For example, in clinical work the aspect of clinical reasoning becomes a method of analysis that may not have been emphasised in years 1 and 2. Whilst in year 3, Tim may need to adapt to this new way of solving clinical problems that may not be fully connected with the content prominence of years 1 and 2. Therefore, the style of learning is likely to be impacted by the learning material required to be learned, and in year 3 there may a distinction in the way material is being taught, which may require a shift in conceptual understanding — a shift from content recollection to reasoning in the practical clinical environment.

5. *Cognitive capability* — Generally we can assume that Tim has no prior issues with cognitive capability and is unlikely to have a learning disability. His newly formed problems with study at year 3 could, however, be linked to issues related to cognitive overload and/or cognitive threshold. Cognitive overload may be an issue with Tim given that he also has problems with time management. Ayres[36] suggested that there are three sources contributing to cognitive overload. First, intrinsic sources may be related to problems with working memory. Second, extraneous sources could be linked to instructional design. Third, germane sources include working memory and the ability to activate schema formulations such as pattern recognition. Cognitive threshold could also be an issue if the learning experiences have changed dramatically thus requiring Tim to adapt to new learning schema, such as moving from content learning to clinical learning, which requires him to work with bedside cases and with 'real patients'.

The Case of Jeanne

Our concerns are:

a) Tends to dominate discussions and had little tolerance towards the opinions of other students

b) Completes most of the tasks on her own even though these tasks were mostly team-based

c) Refuses to accept the feedback from her peers and insists she is the one who always gets things done

Her strengths are:

a) One of the top students and on the Dean's list every year

b) The academic mentor would be meeting with Jeanne to discuss this problem

'Why is Jeanne so Difficult to Handle?'

1. *Emotional and motivational willingness for change* — Jeanne is unlikely to constructively respond to feedback from peers and it is likely that she feels she is coping well.[2] Even though she is unlikely to respond and change after receiving peer feedback, she is likely to be intrinsically robust with a strong sense of self and feels she has no difficulties associated with self-concept, self-efficacy, self-worth and self-determination.[3,37]

   Nonetheless, there is evidence to suggest that she has problems with interpersonal skills, which are crucial when working in medical teams.[4] As a solo act she is perfectly fine but her position may hinder successful completion of complex team-based tasks.[5] The question is 'why' is she so internally focused and negligent of others' needs. In his classic work, Rahim[38] described employees who focused on the communication needs of self rather than others, and suggested these employees could be categorised as having a *dominating* communicating style. He suggested that this forceful approach was often seen when handling differences with juniors than with peers and not at all common when communicating with superiors. When resolving issues there are two possibilities — a concern for one's own goal or a concern for another person's goal — with the optimal communication strategy being to work in the interest of both self and others.[39] Hence, the reason why Jeanne is non-responsive to her peers is probably because she sees them as inferior and, therefore, she is more likely to be responsive to those whom she sees as 'superior'.

2. *Level of academic preparation* — Given her high level of academic attainment (prior and current), it is unlikely that she has any problems academically with coping with the material being studied. Her problem, however, lies in her inability to connect with her peers in a constructive manner. The profession of medicine is essentially about treating people and thus working with people from all walks of life and it is crucial that she is able to communicate with her patients and clinical teams.[8] Her lack of preparation is thus likely in the area of emotional intelligence and social cohesion. The General Medical Council (UK) emphasise the need for doctors to be good, sensitive and effective communicators, which requires them to be responsive and effective listeners.[40] Emotional intelligence may explain 'why' Jeanne finds it

hard to communicate effectively with her peers. Hence, the issue here is not one of academic preparation but of emotional preparation.

3. *Familiarity and expertise with using study enhancement strategies* — From a self-perspective Jeanne has refined effective study skills as she is a top scholar with clear evidence of successful academic attainment. Her problem area is interpersonal integration, which will inevitably cause problems when working in clinical teams. A further issue is the problem of 'disliking', and/or being phobic about the prospect of group work, sometimes referred to as 'grouphate'.[41] Jeanne may not dislike group work but simply sees it as being a hindrance given that she likely perceives herself as being intellectually superior to her peers. She may thus focus more on the disadvantages of group work, such as the need to conform to a majority opinion, that someone may try to dominate her, that it is not time effective, or that she may need to incorporate substandard work done by others.[41] Her reason for dominance may not be about attention-seeking or perceived as being difficult but stems from the fact that she is knowledgeable, able to contribute real insights and solve problems effectively.[42]

4. *Application of learning styles* — As previously discussed her learning preference is to work alone and to dominate discussions. Hence, her learning style may be associated with a competitive approach to learning. Grasha and Yangarber-Hicks[43] proposed that there are six learning styles (competitive, collaborative, avoidant, participant, dependent and independent) and five teaching styles (expert, formal authority, personal model, facilitator and delegator). They further suggest there are several learning styles and the competitive approach embraces the idea of outperforming others to gain greater rewards in the form of greater recognition. She is also utilising a teaching approach more akin to an expert position with an emphasis on showing and transmitting knowledge.

5. *Cognitive capability* — The evidence provided indicates that Jeanne has no issues associated with cognitive capability. The evidence indicated that she excels in her content knowledge and skills, does not appear to be cognitively overloaded or unable to cross a particular cognitive threshold.

Conclusions and Final Thoughts

There is no straightforward answer to the question, 'Why is my student so difficult to handle?' Each student/learner has their own unique set of characteristics and history. Each student/learner has their own reason as to why they find some aspect of the curriculum or a particular teacher difficult to engage with. The causes of such difficulty may lie with the student, learning milieu, teacher and/or the wider environment. To come to terms with the issues at hand requires careful unpacking of all the evidence using a case-by-case strategy. We have used an adapted version of Hirsch's[1] academic counselling framework to illustrate the various components that may contribute to the notion of 'difficulty'.

As Bernstein and Atkinson[44] proposed,

> The reasons why learners struggle are diverse and are often not academic in origin. Moreover, unlike a clinical differential, in which there is usually 1 explanation for the patient's presentation, the struggling learner may be dealing with several issues. Learning is relational; thus, to determine what may be causing problems for a learner ..., it is important to consider what, if any, interactions a student may be having in the learning context that could be interfering with his or her performance. When constructing a differential diagnosis of a learner in difficulty, the acronym 'K-Salts' (knowledge, skills, attitude, learner, teacher, system) is useful. This approach allows the attending to think not only of the skills, attitudes, and behaviours of the learner but also to consider the impact of the environment (p. 210).

Chapter 2: What? — The Tools

In Chapter 1, we considered a framework for diagnosing difficulty. In this chapter, we start to unpack some of the specific tools that faculty staff, counsellors and academic advisors could employ to support learners, especially those perceived as being difficult. We first consider some available tools promoted as being effective and then apply these tools to the same three scenarios we presented in Chapter 1.

University Tools — Programmes and Strategies
Mentoring

Mentoring infers that there is advice from a more experienced learner who could work closely with a less-experienced learner.[45,46] The wise counsel, informational agent or experienced learner is the mentor and the novice learner is the mentee. Mentoring can work at both formal and informal levels. The mentor needs to be experienced in the area of learning, such as medicine, and needs to have an interest in developing the learning of the novice, through listening and imparting ideas, whilst ensuring the relationship is professional, collaborative, authentic and meaningful. The aim is to optimise the full potential of the mentee and assist them in actualising their personal and professional goals.[45]

Mentoring is recognised as a method to assist doctors in their early careers.[47] In their systematic review, Frei and Stamm[45] found that most articles regarding mentoring medical students focussed on career counselling, developing professionalism, supporting personal growth, developing research interests, promoting an academic career and promoting careers in low-interest specialty areas. Mentoring includes both personal and professional facets of development.

Coaching and supervision

In contrast to mentoring, coaching and supervision focuses purely on developing skills.[45] However, similar to mentoring these approaches also draw on informationally rich agents. Hur[48] described a career coaching programme for medical students comprising three facets embedded within a spiral program. The structure embodies the aspects of self-assessment, career planning and career decision making. The career coaching sessions clarify what each student wants, and their corresponding needs as aligned with their career values, which then provides them with a good platform for later development at the specialty level.

Supervision has similar connotations to coaching and a potential definition for supervision[49] with regard to the medical context focuses on the doctor's care of patients. To ensure effective clinical practice, supervision entails providing constructive, timely and accurate feedback based on monitoring performance and encouraging guidance strategies. In the clinical context, emphasis is on patient safety and therefore unambiguous and constructive supervision is imperative when providing essential skills advice.

Feedback systems

In the previous subsection on supervision we mention feedback as being an important component in the process of learning. It is also equally important in mentoring and coaching. There are several components that underlie the feedback process, for example, Nottingham and Henning[50] stated that there are several essential aspects of feedback that include:

- Purpose (confirming or reinforcing behaviour, correcting behaviour and/or promoting improvements for the future)
- Timing (within close proximity to the behaviour)
- Specificity (focusing on actual/observable performance indicators)
- Content (e.g. clinical skills or clinical reasoning)

- Form (using a standardised measurement systems)
- Privacy (using an appropriate setting for giving feedback)

Some overarching themes that make up the feedback process include learning attributes, feedback characteristics and feedback culture.[51] Three key learner characteristics consist of the ability to accurately self-assess one's performance, the ability to take on board feedback and the motivation to want to seek feedback. Feedback characteristics entail the need to improve skills, the type of feedback (multisource, unidirectional and so forth) and the timely nature of feedback. Lastly, it is crucial the institution backs the feedback process and develops a culture for providing constructive feedback regarding workplace performance. In this regard, it is important to develop reliable and valid measurement tools so that feedback systems can accurately appraise performance.

In medical education there are numerous feedback systems and we will mention the different types of feedback techniques cited in the literature[52]:

- Informal systems of feedback occur opportunistically whilst working side by side with the trainee, often at the bedside
- A feedback sandwich that entails giving positive and negative feedback within the confines of a few sentences
- The Pendleton model consisting of four steps: (1) student states what was good about the performance, (2) teacher elaborates on areas of agreement and highlights good performance, (3) student states what could be improved and (4) teacher elaborates on areas that could be improved
- The reflective feedback conversation that emphasises the learner's own ability to self-report the essence of the clinical performance under review

A further refinement of the Pendleton process was mooted by Tan et al.,[53] who suggested the following five-step process when developing effective feedback:

1. Ask the learners what was done well and why (learners' reflections). The aim is to critically revisit the learning process.
2. The teacher will share what was done well and why (teachers' reflection). This is to reinforce students' strengths.
3. Ask the learners what can be done better and how (learners' needs analysis). This is to identify their gaps in learning.
4. The teacher will comment on what can be done better with suggestions for improvement (teachers' needs analysis).
5. Encourage the learners to propose three areas of focus for improvement (action plan) and set a date to review the action plan.

This last technique leads to a discussion about how the performance could be improved. To develop a meaningful approach to feedback that inculcates an effective relationship the term 'education alliance' has surfaced.[54] This alliance infers that teachers and students engage in a two-way conversation where information transfer is negotiated. The key components of this process entail developing a goal consensus and methods for achieving the goal. An alliance is also an important area to develop between peers so that they authentically assess each other.[55]

Reflection

Reflection is a process that often occurs during, or as a product of, the mentoring, coaching or supervision sessions. Sandars[56] proposed that in medical education the approaches that facilitate reflection are:

1. Use of reflective journals
2. Critical incident reports
3. Storytelling

Reflection is considered a meta-cognitive activity (thinking about one's thinking) but also entails an action and planning stage. Reflection can occur at all levels of the process of learning, before, during and after and often entails considering future action based on experiences. Several conceptual models can structure the reflective process. Two of the most commonly cited are Kolb's experiential learning cycle[57] and Gibbs' learning cycle.[58] Both structured models have been applied to the health sciences.

The reflective cycle presented by Kolb suggested there are four dimensions[56] that include:

1. Concrete experience or what happened?
2. Reflective observation or analysis
3. Abstract conceptualisation or making generalisations
4. Active experimentation planning future action

Gibbs'[58] cycle has the following six components:

1. Based on description (what happened?)
2. Feelings (what were you thinking and feeling?)
3. Evaluation (what was good and bad about the experience?)
4. Analysis (what sense can you make of the situation?)
5. Conclusion (what else could you have done?)
6. Action plan (if it arose again what would you do?).

As we can see, these two reflective cycles are very similar; nevertheless, they allow us to structure and focus the reflective process leading to a tangible and attainable outcome.

Sandars[56] suggested that educational strategies need to be structured to optimise the process of reflection. First, we need to ensure students are motivated to engage in reflection such that it is important to consider the role of intrinsic motivation, self-efficacy and ease at which a task can be completed. Extrinsic motivation likely plays a role and assessment will often drive student learning or engagement. Second, is how to develop the meta-cognitive skills for reflection, such as noticing, processing and developing future plans.[53] In developing the skills of noticing it is important to promote self-monitoring and the willingness to hear and see feedback, and to notice critical incidents. Processing skills can be developed through promoting reflection for learning, for enhancing a therapeutic relationship and for improving professional expertise. Developing one's future necessitates recognition of learning needs that are aligned with developing an achievable plan.

Academic and personal counselling

Providing academic and personal counselling services within a medical school is becoming more commonplace. For example, Gaughf and Foster[59] described these services as institutionally sanctioned with a focus on students experiencing academic and/or personal difficulty. In Chapter 1, we introduced Hirsch's idea of diagnosing the areas of difficulty experienced by students.[1] Academic and personal counsellor roles may overlap, with the main overlapping responsibility to assess level and type of difficulty so that the most appropriate assistance is provided, thus ensuring optimal academic and personal success for the student. Gaughf et al.[59] stated that crucial skills are:

1. Addressing the transitioning process between years of study within a university programme
2. Gaining study skills and personal assessment through evaluating grade achievement, using established measures and/or gaining qualitative information
3. Developing time management and organisational skills
4. Reviewing and optimising test and assessment strategies
5. Clarifying career and academic goals and interests
6. Increasing self-confidence and coping with self-doubt
7. Coping and managing mental health issues, such as depression and/or anxiety

8. Developing stress management tools
9. Working with relationship issues and developing conflict management skills
10. Working through loss and bereavement

Motivational and self-regulatory learning strategies are key to any successful intervention. Motivation is a large area of research that encompasses many theories. These can include theories related to behaviour, cognition, psychoanalysis, humanism, social learning and social cognition. Weinstein and Palmer[34] stated that areas of learning can be broken down into three components: skill, will and self-regulation. Skill is related to information processing, selection of main ideas and test-taking strategies. Will is connected to motivation and emotion. Self-regulation involves meta-cognition components, such as planning, monitoring and modifying skill behaviour. It also aims to appraise and enhance areas linked to concentration, self-testing, study aids and time management.

In Chapter 1, we referred to the idea of the open arena and blind spot. Halpern[28] suggested that academic counsellors and their clients can explore the 'open arena' to establish common ground with the intent to build up trust and provide a means to engender change. The counsellors could develop ground rules that are acceptable to both parties and set an agenda that can lead to transformative action. Halpern[28] suggested that the blind spot issue needs to be addressed in line with the context and the information gleaned from probing into the academic and non-academic life surrounding students in difficulty. Counsellors could begin by asking students for options for change rather than explicitly providing solutions. They could also apply the modified version of Pendleton's approach by incorporating Tan et al.'s[53] refinement.

Learning contracts

Learning contracts are documents and systems that formalise the supervision, mentoring or coaching processes. Teachers and students usually sign the document and the expectations are agreed on, although the creation of such a document may be difficult to enact and generate due to brief encounters between key stakeholders. Nevertheless, some of the criteria agreed on include the material or skills that are to be learned, how this process of learning is to be conducted and how the learning will be verified or assessed.[60] To be successful, learning contracts need to be self-directed and self-initiated. Similar to any learning process the key elements of the learning contract are the learning objectives, the resources available, the strategies to use these resources and evidence that learning has occurred.[60]

Individual Responsibilities

Career trajectory and intrinsic interest

Career trajectory and intrinsic interest have an individual focus but can also be assisted by the factors considered above. In medicine, students often have short- and long-term goals, and as they progress through their education they begin to have firmer ideas about which discipline they would like to work in. For example, Puertas and Arósquipa[61] found that certain intrinsic factors were able to more firmly predict which medical students in South America had a more defined idea of a career in primary care. These factors were income status, being married or older, and a positive social attitude towards those in less-privileged populations. Hence, the proximity in terms of self (as clinician) and other (prospective patients) will influence the motivation of medical students and their career intention.

There is also some evidence that interest in the altruistic desire to help patients motivated doctors to take up a career in primary care.[61] Interactions with and influences from the medical school environment also played a role in career intention.[61] In addition, student interest is also moderated by their need to succeed especially in the immediate sense with regard to task completion (passing their course) and in the longer term as clinicians who want to develop their professional and academic careers.[62]

Exercise and well-being strategies

Students and clinicians in their early careers are often at loggerheads with coping with their stressful learning and working environments.[26,27] There are many strategies that early career students could employ to become more resilient and to promote their well-being. Some strategies are linked to the development of the learning environment and the curriculum within that environment.[63] One key consideration is the notion of the coping reservoir, which includes harnessing the family and social support networks, especially as many meaningful friendships are cultivated whilst at university.[63] The reservoir can be depleted in competitive learning environments, when career options become limited and when students fail to seek help as it may be interpreted as a 'loss of face' especially amongst Asian students and this is a problem especially amongst international students who lack easy access to family and close friend networks.[64]

Minimising the risk of burnout often requires students and early career clinicians to reach out to those personally closest to them (e.g. friends), although if the issue is more akin to their professional role then they need to reach out to mentors, teachers and trusted seniors. There are also numerous self-help systems that could be accessed to promote well-being and minimise the risk of adverse problems. For example, Moir et al.[65] developed and researched help-seeking behaviours associated with students accessing a website for medical students that contains useful material that can assist them during their learning years. This CALM (Computer Assisted Learning for the Mind) website[66] provides information and material to address the areas of:

1. Mental resilience
2. Managing stress, anxiety and depression
3. Healthy relationships
4. Finding meaning in life

Applying These Strategies to the Case Scenarios Presented In Chapter 1

The case of Peter (resident)

In Peter's case, using Hirsch's (1) diagnosis criteria, there are several potential causes to the issues presented that could be addressed using the above strategies (see summary in Table 1).

We have identified several issues that may explain why Peter is perceived as being difficult. The more accurate the diagnostic phase the clearer the solution will be. To create some order in creating an intervention, we need to converge our assumptions with the facts at hand by first considering previous strategies to deal with similar student problems, then forming a theoretical approach to deal with the main issues and thereby backing this up with existing evidence and ongoing observational data.[67] We need to start with the most obvious point of entry, which appears to be the inability to receive feedback effectively, thus impairing a level of self-awareness and a willingness to change (Fig. 1).

Figure 1 indicates an interlinked approach to addressing the issues raised in Peter's case, by first starting with strategy 1 'Increasing awareness (thinking and emotional well-being)' and then working through to strategies 2 and 3. Therefore, we believe that the type of intervention that would likely yield the greatest chance of success is to begin with developing systems to promote awareness and the willingness for change. This would likely require the assignment of a mentor, whose task is to work with Peter and to begin with developing his communication and professionalism skills so that he is able to receive and work on the feedback being given to him. If successful, this will likely enable entry into developing systems to tackle first professional and affective issues (time management and well-being), and then consider strategies for cognitive development (developing deep learning approaches and knowledge consolidation). It is hypothesised that the mentor will have to be respected by

Table 1. The case of Peter: Diagnostic foci, main issues identified and potential solutions.

Potential diagnostic component identified	Main issues	Solutions
Emotional and motivational willingness to change	Unwilling to accept shortcomings, potential blind spot, block in open arena, communication issues	Mentoring, coaching or close supervision
	Potential problems with well-being and balance	Academic and personal counselling
Level of academic preparation	Knowledge gaps	Developing feedback systems regarding cognitive strategies with action points
Use of study enhancement strategies	Time management (meta-cognitive) problems	Development of meta-cognitive strategies
	Cognitive issues	Developing cognitive strategies, e.g. memory, reasoning
Application of learning styles	Using a surface rather deep learning approach	Strategies to encourage deep learning
Cognitive capability	Potential learning disability, attention related problem or mental illness	Further psychological assessment, which may require referral
	Potential cognitive overload	Focussing on what needs to be learnt
	Inability to meet the required cognitive threshold	Mentoring, coaching or close supervision

Peter and be experienced, knowledgeable, empathetic and reflective.[45–47] The questions that need to be answered are, why is the 'open arena' dysfunctional and what are the 'blind spots'?

Given the issues with knowledge and time management a formalised mentoring system needs to be instigated (with a learning contract in place) so that Peter is more motivated to be engaged with the process. The mentor will need to document progress and challenges being faced by Peter in case a further referral to an academic and personal counsellor is required. The academic and personal counsellor will have systems in place to offer a more detailed psychological/educational assessment that can be used to assist with Peter's further development, such as dealing with lifestyle balance, cognitive overload and overcoming cognitive thresholds.

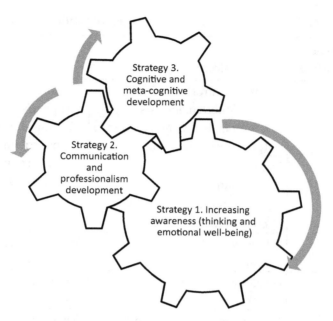

Fig. 1.   Relationships between evidence and skill development.

The case of Tim (third-year medical student)

We have tackled Tim's case, using a similar process to that described above, although his issues are contextually and situationally unique. His main issues relate to being late when coming to class and submitting assignments, keeping very quiet during class discussions and his grades had been falling over the past semester. The several hypothesised causes to the issues presented are addressed using the above strategies (Table 2).

We have identified several issues (Table 2) that may explain why Tim is perceived as being difficult. First, a more detailed diagnostic picture needs to be developed and this could be conducted by the Module Co-ordinator and then by a mentor, coach or supervisor. Mentoring is likely to be less intrusive and the first thing to try in Tim's case. The Module Co-ordinator will need to appraise which referral mechanism will have the greatest chance of success. If Tim is in need of psychological intervention then an academic and/or personal counsellor needs to be contacted. If Tim's needs are appraised as being caught in a temporary state of inertia due to lack of support then a mentor may be the more appropriate place to start.

Figure 2 suggests strategies for dealing with Tim's issues, beginning with clarifying 'Motivation for studying medicine and emotional preparedness for Year 3' then moving to strategies 2 and 3. In Tim's case, it would be useful for the Module Co-ordinator to appraise his willingness for further study and his ability to cope with the emotional demands of early clinical work. If the Module Co-ordinator feels that Tim is isolated then a mentoring

Table 2.   The case of Tim: Diagnostic foci, main issues identified and potential solutions.

Potential diagnostic component identified	Main issues	Solutions
Emotional and motivational willingness to change	Locus of control — internal (self-doubt/anxiousness, emotionally distant) or external (pressures from family)	Mentoring, coaching or close supervision Working with families and close friends (if appropriate) to ascertain the quality of existing social networks
	Stability — Can he change or not change?	
	Controllability — Is he able to control the situation?	
Level of academic preparation	Adapting to the new curriculum and knowledge	Analysing his achievements and non-achievements.
Use of study enhancement strategies	Grades are falling	Development of cognitive strategies
	Lateness when coming to class	Developing meta-cognitive strategies through using effective feedback systems
Application of learning styles	Failing to adapt to new ways of learning. Is the knowledge difficult or the clinical work or both?	Mentoring and academic counselling
Cognitive capability	Potential Learning disability, attention-related problem or mental illness	Further psychological assessment, which may require referral
	Potential cognitive overload	Focussing on his ability to cope
	Inability to meet the required cognitive threshold	Close supervision and academic counselling

intervention is likely a good place to start. If the mentor finds that Tim is struggling with the new knowledge level then an academic counsellor needs to be consulted so that cognitive strategies can be put in place (i.e. developing reasoning skills). If the early clinical exposure is causing problems then a more personalized approach using a personal counsellor or psychologist may need to be approached. Finally, once these early stages are investigated then addressing lateness and a commitment to be involved in class discussions will likely be straightforward and if persistent may require a learning contract.

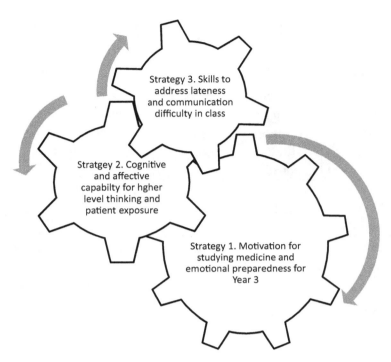

Fig. 2.   Relationships between evidence and skill development.

The case of Jeanne (medical student)

As with Peter and Tim, we have some evidence regarding Jeanne's level of difficulty. Her main issues are dominating discussions with little tolerance towards others, completes most team-based tasks on her own and refuses to accept the feedback from her peers. Using Hirsch's[1] diagnostic framework we have suggested some key issues with several hypothesised strategies (Table 3).

Figure 3 illustrates our integrated approach to dealing with the issues raised in Jeanne's case starting with strategy 1 and then moving to 2 and 3. In Jeanne's case, the most evident problem is being able to constructively work with peers. Hence, it is likely that a senior mentor or supervisor needs to first work with Jeanne to develop her social and workplace awareness with a particular focus on developing responsiveness to peers (Fig. 3). Being responsive to peer feedback is one of the major learning processes that can be useful for professional development. Next, a more specific strategy could be developed to address Jeanne's inability to work in teams and to heighten her reflection skills. One area that could be addressed is creating Jeanne's involvement and commitment to work in a team-based culture so that peers are able to assess each other in a honest and cordial learning environment.[55] Reflection skills can be developed using established models, such as Kolb's and Gibbs' models of reflection.[57,58]

Table 3. The case of Jeanne: Diagnostic foci, main issues identified and potential solutions.

Potential diagnostic components identified	Main issues	Solutions
Emotional and motivational willingness to change	Unresponsive to feedback from peers	It is likely a supervisor or senior mentor (someone she looks up to) will have more influence than a peer mentor
	Perceptions that she is always right and thus unwilling change	
	Negligent of others' needs — dominant communicative style	
Level of academic preparation	Emotional intelligence issues and problems in developing social cohesion	Senior mentor or supervisor can work on developing social and workplace interaction and reflecting on the value of others' opinions
Use of study enhancement strategies	Dislikes group work or working in teams	Senior mentor or supervisor needs to highlight the importance of clinical team work Use of meta-cognitive feedback, such as developing a need's analysis with Jeanne along with a viable action plan
Application of learning styles	Prefers to work alone and highly competitive	As above — also need to work with the positives and negatives of being overly competitive
Cognitive capability	No issues identified	NA

Finally, on the same theme, more specific skills need to be addressed such as Jeanne's preponderance for being dominant, which could be transformed to leadership. In addition, a leadership role may enable her to cultivate a more responsive approach to competitiveness.

Concluding Comments

In this chapter, we have provided some strategies (tools) that could be refined to address difficulty issues related to medical students and early career doctors. We have built on the diagnostic approaches provided in Chapter 1 and applied these ideas and strategies to the, formerly described, three student scenarios. Clearly, the difficulty issues could be addressed by starting at a generic level and then focusing more on skill development. Trying to convince

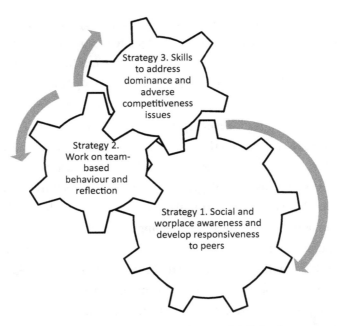

Fig. 3.   Relationships between evidence and skill development.

students to change and be responsive to feedback is one of the challenges of medical teachers and academic counsellors. Once students and professionals become more receptive to feedback and reflective practice then the issues of change become more about skill development. To initiate this change process requires informational agents (mentors, supervisors, and coaches) to work with junior professionals to optimise the opportunity for change.

Chapter 3: How?

In Chapters 1 and 2, we have reviewed aspects of difficulty from diagnostic perspectives as well as considering targeted interventions. Accordingly, we have determined possible reasons as to why a student may be perceived as being difficult or act in a disruptive manner, and ways in which this behaviour could be ameliorated. In this chapter, we consider 'how' wider implications are addressed in relation to student support and institutional responsibilities. More specifically, we focus on university guidelines, ethical and moral issues, and the notion of the psychological contract.

University Guidelines and Policies

Most universities have a set of guidelines on appropriate behaviour. Guidelines and regulations regarding academic misconduct are often clearly stated and focus on behaviour associated with course completion and penalties for dishonest engagement. They form the legal standpoint from which the university operates, whereas agencies of justice resolve criminal behaviour beyond the statutes. Within the university context, transgression from the academic code of conduct are met with penalties with severity dependent upon the magnitude of the transgression.

University behaviour policies are established to demarcate appropriate behavioural expectations. For example, at the University of Tasmania,[68] a document was produced to set out the values, standards and expectations for appropriate behaviour within this university. The values set out include respect for colleagues, self and the learning environment, and the promotion of 'fairness and justice, integrity, trust and trustworthiness, responsibility and honesty (p. 3)'.[68] The University of Tasmania document also endorses the importance of interpersonal relationships, managing and respecting difference, and encouraging speaking up protocols. Unacceptable conduct can include disruptive behaviour, unlawful discrimination, harassment and bullying, vilification and sexual misconduct. If unacceptable behaviour is witnessed or experienced, the University of Tasmania have put in place a system to deal with such behaviours, such as promoting disclosure, developing a complaints procedure, encouraging involvement of the police or external agencies (especially when criminal activity is witnessed or experienced), providing contact details for 'behaviour contact officers' and clearly setting out university policies.

Similarly, codes of conduct are documents that clearly define expected standards for staff and students. For example, the University of Alberta[69] has created a document defining 'unacceptable behaviour for Students in the University, the sanctions for commission of the offences, and explanations of the complete discipline and appeal processes (p. 2)'.[69] Inappropriate behaviour includes engaging in plagiarism, cheating, misuse of confidential materials, research and scholarship misconduct; inappropriate behaviour in professional programs; inappropriate action towards individuals or groups; violations of safety or dignity; and inappropriate use of university property and resources. Types of sanctions that could be applied include conduct probation, encumbrance, exclusion, expulsion, fines, grade reductions, rescission of admittance or a degree, restitution, reprimand and suspension. At the University of Alberta,[69] disciplinary decisions are subjected to a sanctioned process including alerting students to the general rules of discipline and appeal, service and notice, a complaints procedure and procedures for disciplinary officers and Deans.

Medical schools require a further inspection of professional conduct. For example, the Duke University School of Medicine[70] have developed a document that aims to promote engagement in intellectual integrity and honesty in all endeavours, the need for the concern for the welfare of others, respect for the rights of others and the need to promote professional demeanour and behaviour. Some of the professionally focused behaviours promoted at this university comprise learning '...to recognize when his/her ability to function effectively is compromised, ask for relief or help, and notify the responsible person if something interferes with the ability to perform clinical or research tasks safely and effectively (p. 2)'.[70]

In the medical education context, there are important reasons for managing students with difficulty or dealing with students who are struggling. In their systematic review, Frellsen et al.[71] 'sought to characterize the policies of U.S. and Canadian medical schools regarding struggling medical students during the core internal medicine clerkship and fourth-year internal medicine rotations (p. 876)'. They found that from 83 institutions the reported percentage of struggling students varied considerably from between 0% and 23% of students. The crucial part of any policy requirement was to have institutional mechanisms identifying students who are struggling and support systems in place to remediate these students.

Policies regarding identification are critically important and this becomes more important when the potential implications of malpractice are present. Identifying and characterising medical students with difficulty, and those who present as being difficult, is of critical importance in medical education and if left unchecked can lead to major problems later on such as compromised patient care.[71] One clear example of identifying students who are struggling is to have systems in place to continuously audit students' grade achievements, such as was the case for Tim in our case scenarios. In this case scenario, cited in Chapters 1 and 2, Tim's grades had been falling over the semester, even though he had very good grades in his first and second years. This alerted university personnel to investigate further.

Several further implications at the university level are highlighted in the literature. For example, Frellsen et al.[71] reported that students struggling with achievement were sent to a school committee rather than a 'module coordinator', as was the case for Tim. One of the roles of a school committee is to make decisions regarding student advancement given their indicated level of difficulty. In Tim's case, his grade scores are clear evidence of non-achievement or a trend indicating academic dysfunction. A major consideration for Tim's case is the implication for procedural and distributive justice. Lizzio and Wilson[72] found that students constructed their perception of fairness based on a respectful partnership between themselves and university staff and having faith that there is systemic fairness inbuilt within the university policy. Accordingly, decisions are based on a fair and considered process suggesting that Tim would likely be more responsive to change if he felt the university were vested in his success as a student, by showing responsive support for his need to succeed. The ethical dilemma that can occur relates to the need for justice for the student as well as considering the impact on the university and, in the case of medical education, future care for patients. There is also the university responsibility regarding their ultimate mandate to produce competent graduates.[73]

Colbert et al.[74] investigated the issue of fairness as it relates to decisions made regarding student behaviour. Using a systems' lens they examined the application and concept of fairness as it applies to postgraduate medical education contexts. The decisions based around 'what to do with difficult students' needs to include discussions relating to educational opportunities, assessment practices and the context of the learning environment. In Chapters 1 and 2, three student scenarios were presented to illustrate certain problematic behaviours. Peter has problems with content knowledge and time management. As discussed, Tim has difficulties with maintaining his grade point average, which is accompanied with being withdrawn in class. Jeanne has difficulties with working with peers and being tolerant of others' opinions. In all cases, the problem has not yet reached decisions requiring legal action. And hence, the university position is clear regarding implementation of in-house strategies such as those suggested in Chapter 2.

Nevertheless, the issue of fairness is worthy of further mention, given that judgements are being made regarding Peter and Tim's level of competency. Equity or fairness in assessment practices is based on the assumption that, all things being equal, each trainee has access to comparable opportunities to learn and subsequently assessment can differentiate between the attainment of knowledge and skills between students with the consideration of their unique backgrounds.[74] With interventions being applied, as mentioned in Chapters 1 and 2, we can envisage that all students (Peter, Tim and Jeanne) will have opportunities to redress any potential gaps in learning, whether this be knowledge, time management or communication.

Ethical and Moral Responsibilities

Ethical and moral responsibilities are linked to the individual and the university.

The individual

As they get closer to certification, a medical student has a professional obligation to be competent, which requires ongoing attention, life-long learning, and this is linked to the need to harness ethical and moral responsibilities. Professional duty as linked with ethical and moral responsibilities is the backbone of the medical vocation and has significant attitudinal components. For example, we noted that self-care issues may be related to some of the students' difficulties found in the scenarios cited in Chapters 1 and 2 (i.e. Peter, Tim and Jeanne). It has been asserted that self-care concerns for medical students is common place in the literature, such as those related to gaining appropriate nutrition, engaging in exercise routines and creating wellbeing goals.[75]

Pellegrino[76] further proposes that the essence of being a professional, which is an assumption made regarding medical student and junior residents' behaviour, is a statement that supports and respects the public good and implicit in this position is a commitment and dedication to an ideal, such as being the best doctor they can be. According to Pellegrino, the act of being a professional in medicine is linked to two factors. The first occurs when a graduate makes a solemn and public promise when the 'Hippocratic Oath' is taken to enter into a contract with the institution that they have now completed a degree in medicine and as such become a medical professional, and part of this rite of passage is going from student to graduated medical professional. The second aspect is about practice and the assumptions based around interaction with patients, who they will likely see on a daily basis. The manifestation of doctor–patient interaction implies that they are present and competent for the patient good.

In their debate regarding the relevance of the Hippocratic Oath to the ethical and moral values of contemporary medicine, Askitopoulou and Vgontzas[77] stated, 'The Hippocratic Oath for the first time defined a moral code for medical behaviour and distinguished professional expertise from personal morality in medicine (p. 1483)'. This succinct statement and promise extends beyond the self-interest of the professional to include the needs of patient and responsibilities associated with patient care. As such,

> The Oath conveys the duties and commitments of a physician to the best interest of the patient. It establishes the general moral conduct of the physician–patient relationship, which reflects long lasting ethical values that still govern the medical profession. The Oath introduces the principles of beneficence, non-maleficence and confidentiality and asks for accountability from the medical community (p. 1483).[77]

The implications of the 'Oath' are that once graduated the medical professional proclaims that they now have specialist knowledge, which can be used as a skill to promote and enact optimal patient care. At this stage they enter into not only a professional community but also a moral community aimed at advancing the welfare of patients.[76] There is also an implied consideration for the individual to engage in meta-cognition and, thus, be reflective and seek feedback at regular intervals.[53] Askitopoulou and Vgontzas[77] further state,

> An oath is a solemn voluntary pledge usually invoking a divine witness; it is the declaration of a principle and a guarantee of the oath taker's trustworthiness, binding the individual personally. A code is a collection of injunctions and

prohibitions, usually created by an authoritative body to provide comprehensive standards for the practicing decision-maker (p. 1485).

In reference to the three scenarios presented in Chapters 1 and 2, there are several ramifications. Tim and Jeanne have yet to make the oath whilst Peter is a resident and thus practicing during his clerkship. Nevertheless, the implication is clear that for Tim, Peter and Jeanne the need to achieve maximal competency is of paramount importance. By entering into a university that teaches medicine, these three students are proclaiming an intention to uphold the 'Oath' as practicing future and present professionals. Therefore, they have a responsibility to reflect on their competencies with an intention to develop and remediate any defects of practice.

The university

The learning experiences of students are underscored by the teaching provided within universities. Students perceive that teachers have certain professional obligations linked with the educational strategies of universities. In the pursuit of students' opinions regarding the students' expectations of teacher knowledge, skills and attitudes as linked to intrinsic or a more inclusive meaning of education, Semradova and Hubackova[78] provide a list of professional features that students feel would ensure the pedagogical process is responsible and competent. The list requires to teachers to:

- have professional knowledge
- be goal-directed
- utilise a recognised and effective pedagogical approach
- possess psychological and methodological knowledge
- be able to respond to impulses from students
- have a knowledge of the legal boundaries, competency requirements and responsibilities
- be able to motivate pupils or students
- possess facets of self-control
- be adaptable to various situations and be creative
- possess authority and be able to handle topics from a professional, factual and methodological point of view
- be precise, disciplined and a critical thinker
- be active regarding team work development
- activate deep learning
- be involved with careful preparation
- be engaged in their own scientific activity

In addition to this list, Semradova and Hubackova[78] present a student inventory related to communication expectations that include:

- using appropriate verbal and non-verbal tools
- providing clear presentations and tasks
- ensuring there is bidirectionality of the communication activity
- encouraging debates, dialogues and discussions
- allowing space for written expression
- having tolerance of different opinions
- paying attention to all students
- engaging in fair assessment
- utilising appropriate information and communications technology

Blaskova et al.[79] also suggest that universities need to be competent in themselves as an organisation. A key aspect of competence is related to the notion of success, which in university terms relates to academic achievement and scholarly research-based outputs. In their article, the theme of Universities functioning as a competent entity is discussed in terms of universities:

- dealing with and promoting teaching innovations
- ensuring the development of teachers
- auditing and promoting learning development
- actively connecting teaching and scholarship
- dealing with knowledge and knowledge management
- being responsible
- dealing with constructivism in Universities' and teachers' action
- ensuring competences of teachers
- employing quality control systems

Self-care issues and those related to well-being have a definite crossover between individual and institutional responsibility.[75] At the University of Auckland, the school of medicine have embedded a core curricula strand dealing with well-being and professionalism issues.[80] In their paper, Ayala et al.[75] further stated that many institutions have formal programmes embedded within the curricula to address well-being concerns, for example, physical and mental health. Nonetheless, they suggest that even though these programmes have been shown to be effective, they could be more optimally applied if they included 'the opinions of medical students regarding which self-care, health promotion, and burnout prevention, activities are most useful to them (p. 243)'.[75]

The main drivers of the university are located in management, overseeing financial, infrastructure and human resources perspectives. Departments catering to student affairs are also critical to universities. Therefore, universities have a responsibility to satisfy students and the communities they serve and to create resource development to ensure learning is optimized.[81] Universities are responsible for procuring students who are competent and fit for the requirements of their profession. In any educational course, the standard of competency is established by creating fair and valid assessment protocols. In medical education, the assessment protocols tend to be complex and multi-layered. Assessment within a medical education context is linked to the development of learning objectives and reasonable exposure to teaching and learning activities.[82] It is not the purpose of this chapter to review the concept of assessment within education, but it is important that student competencies are determined by performance on assessments and the assumptions are that these assessments are authentic, reliable, discriminatory and valid mechanisms.

Returning to the scenarios — What are the responsibilities of the university? Tim, Peter and Jeanne have been classified as being difficult. Hence, the responsibility of the university is to first check that their management and teaching processes are functioning optimally before attributing blame towards the students. It is likely that many parties have to engage in some reflection and learning and as such both the organisation [university] and the students learn.[83]

The psychological contract

Koskina[84] has put forward a convincing argument to suggest that the psychological contract has direct relevance for engagement within the higher education context. Higher education, including medical schools, has undergone major structural and functional changes in recent decades. One of the major changes relates to the market economy and the business model, which often motivates and creates the framework for the successful operation of higher education institutions. With the advent of the business model comes the need to compete with other institutions for funding and student enrolments, which influences tuition fees and university financing priorities.

Within this market economy, students become more aligned as customers than learners per se.[85] According to this shift in priorities, students have definite expectations of what they should be purchasing and teachers are required to ensure the customer is satisfied.[86] In this educational–business ambience, the psychological contract becomes very important and relates to stratifying how the university can manage the difficulties arising for the three scenarios previously discussed (Tim, Peter and Jeanne). The psychological contract relates to individual beliefs and expectations associated with a perceived exchange agreement between the university and students.[84]

One facet of expectation relates to students' perceptions of value or literally 'value-for-money'. Students will come into a course with preconceived notions of what is of value and what they need to learn. They also have perceptions of what is interesting and what lecturers need to do to make their lessons interesting.[86] This impacts not only the delivery of information, but also its assessment and the learning outcomes that the lessons are based on. An area of medical education influencing student satisfaction is feedback.[87] Boehler et al.[87] found that students' satisfaction was more related to the use of 'compliments' than feedback for learning in this randomised controlled trial. The compliment group gave significantly higher ratings than the feedback group, even though the feedback group had gained more informational instruction.

When applying the psychological contact to Tim, Peter and Jeanne, we can hypothesise that the barriers to students' learning and autonomy are linked to the notion of what should be taught and provided by the university. Jeanne has definite beliefs around the value of the informational provider and sees her peers as lower than her cognitively rich 'superiors', and therefore, her psychological contract is that her learning needs to be directed by superiors rather than peers. This thinking has some logic but will likely impede her teamwork behaviour once working on the wards and may lead to comprised patient care. Peter has worrying shortcomings, but his psychological contract may suggest to him that it is the institution's responsibility to educate him and that he is paying high fees for this service. This may be blocking any possibility of taking responsibility for his learning and developing as an autonomous life-long learner, which is one of the ideals of the developing doctor.[88] In the case of Tim, his psychological contract may be perceived as the receiver of information and he has yet to comprehend that it is sometimes just as important to give as to receive.

Final Thoughts

In this section, we have concentrated on three chapters related to the idea of 'what to do when faced with difficult students?' We began by diagnosing the issues then offering some professional interventions, and finally considering the wider picture by including the institutional obligations, policies and guidelines. It is likely that there can be some generic strategies for working with students perceived as being difficult, but ultimately the stories are likely to be unique requiring case-by-case approaches and analysis.

References

1. Hirsch G. *Helping College Students Succeed: A Model for Effective Intervention*. Mineapolis: Brunner-Routledge; 2001.

2. Marroquín B, Tennen H, Stanton AL. Coping, emotion regulation, and well-being: Intrapersonal and interpersonal processes. In: Robinson MD, Eid M, editors. *The Happy Mind: Cognitive Contributions to Well-Being*. Springer; 2017:253–74.

3. Schunk DH, DiBenedetto MK. Self-efficacy theory in education. In: Wentzel KR, Miele DB, editors. *Handbook of Motivation at School*. 2nd ed. New York: Routledge; 2016:34–54.

4. Türel YK. Relationships between students' perceived team learning experiences, team performances, and social abilities in a blended course setting. *The Internet and Higher Education*. 2016;31:79–86.

5. Mao A, Mason W, Suri S, Watts DJ. An experimental study of team size and performance on a complex task. *PloS One*. 2016;11(4):e0153048.

6. Bluteau P, Clouder L, Cureton D. Developing interprofessional education online: An ecological systems theory analysis. *Journal of Interprofessional Care*. 2017;31(4):420–8.

7. Scicluna HA, O'Sullivan AJ, Boyle P, Jones PD, McNeil HP. Peer learning in the UNSW Medicine program Assessment and evaluation of admissions, knowledge, skills and attitudes. *BMC Medical Education*. 2015;15:167-1-167-9.

8. Careau E, Biba G, Brander R, Van Dijk JP, Verma S, Paterson M, et al. Health leadership education programs, best practices, and impact on learners' knowledge, skills, attitudes, and behaviors and system change: A literature review. *Journal of Healthcare Leadership*. 2014;6:39–50.

9. Pintrich PR. A motivational science perspective on the role of student motivation in learning and teaching contexts. *Journal of Educational Psychology*. 2003;95(4):667.

10. Weinstein C, Acee TW. Study and learning strategies. In: Flippo RF, Bean TW, editors. *Handbook of College Reading and Study Strategy Research*. 3rd ed. New York: Routledge; 2018:227–40.

11. Sandars J, Cleary TJ. Self-regulation theory: Applications to medical education: AMEE Guide No. 58. *Medical Teacher*. 2011;33(11):875–86.

12. Norman G. Data dredging, salami-slicing, and other successful strategies to ensure rejection: Twelve tips on how to not get your paper published. *Advances in Health Sciences Education*. 2014;19:1–5.

13. Newble D, Entwistle N. Learning styles and approaches: Implications for medical education. *Medical Education*. 1986;20(3):162–75.

14. Zhu H-r, Zeng H, Zhang H, Zhang H-y, Wan F-j, Guo H-h, et al. The preferred learning styles utilizing VARK among nursing students with bachelor degrees and associate degrees in China. *Acta Paulista de Enfermagem*. 2018;31(2):162–9.

15. Biggs J. What do inventories of students' learning processes really measure? A theoretical review and clarification. *British Journal of Educational Psychology*. 1993;63(1):3–19.

16. Abdelhamid TM. The multidimensional learning model: A novel cognitive psychology-based model for computer assisted instruction in order to improve learning in medical students. *Medical Education Online*. 1999;4(1):4302.

17. Zywno MS, Waalen JK. The effect of individual learning styles on student outcomes in technology-enabled education. *Global Journal of Engineering Education Australia*. 2002;6(1):35–44.

18. Rosebraugh CJ. Learning disabilities and medical schools. *Medical Education*. 2000;34(12):994–1000.

19. Heiman T, Precel K. Students with learning disabilities in higher education: Academic strategies profile. *Journal of Learning Disabilities*. 2003;36(3):248–58.

20. Young JQ, Van Merrienboer J, Durning S, Ten Cate O. Cognitive load theory: Implications for medical education: AMEE guide no. 86. *Medical Teacher*. 2014;36(5):371–84.

21. Barr DA. Science as superstition: Selecting medical students. *The Lancet*. 2010;376(9742):678–9.

22. Flanagan M. Threshold concepts: Undergraduate teaching, postgraduate training, professional development and school education. A short introduction and a bibliograph; 2018. Available from: https://www.ee.ucl.ac.uk/~mflanaga/thresholds.html.

23. Wearn A, O'Callaghan A, Barrow M. Becoming a different doctor: Identifying threshold concepts when doctors in training spend six months with a hospital palliative care team. In: Land R, Meyer JHF, Flanagan MT, editors. *Threshold Concepts in Practice*. Rotterdam: Sense Publishers; 2016:223–38.

24. Specialists Accreditation Board. Graduate Medical Education in Singapore Singapore: Ministry of Health; 2018. Available from: http://www.healthprofessionals.gov.sg/sab/specialist-training/graduate-medical-education-in-singapore.

25. Pereira-Lima K, Loureiro S. Burnout, anxiety, depression, and social skills in medical residents. *Psychology, Health & Medicine*. 2015;20(3):353–62.

26. Dyrbye LN, Shanafelt T. A narrative review on burnout experienced by medical students and residents. *Medical Education*. 2016;50(1):132–49.

27. Henning MA, Hawken SJ, Hill AG. The quality of life of New Zealand doctors and medical students: What can be done to avoid burnout? *The New Zealand Medical Journal*. 2009;122(1307):102–10.

28. Halpern H. Supervision and the Johari window: A framework for asking questions. *Education for Primary Care*. 2009;20(1):10–14.

29. White SM, Riley A, Flom P. Assessment of Time Management Skills (ATMS): A practice-based outcome questionnaire. *Occupational Therapy in Mental Health*. 2013;29(3):215–31.

30. Dolmans DH, Loyens SM, Marcq H, Gijbels D. Deep and surface learning in problem-based learning: A review of the literature. *Advances in Health Sciences Education*. 2016;21(5):1087–112.

31. Broadbent J, Poon W. Self-regulated learning strategies & academic achievement in online higher education learning environments: A systematic review. *The Internet and Higher Education*. 2015;27:1–13.

32. Weiner B. An attributional theory of achievement motivation and emotion. *Psychological Review*. 1985;92(4):548–73.

33. Genn J. AMEE Medical Education Guide No. 23 (Part 1): Curriculum, environment, climate, quality and change in medical education — a unifying perspective. *Medical Teacher*. 2001;23(4):337–44.

34. Weinstein C, Palmer D. *LASSI-HS User's Manual*. 2nd ed. Clearwater, FL: H & H Publishing Company, Inc; 1990.

35. Billett S. Learning through health care work: Premises, contributions and practices. *Medical Education.* 2016;50(1):124–31.

36. Ayres P. Using subjective measures to detect variations of intrinsic cognitive load within problems. *Learning and Instruction.* 2006;16(5):389–400.

37. Evans P. Self-determination theory: An approach to motivation in music education. *Musicae Scientiae.* 2015;19(1):65–83.

38. Rahim MA. A measure of styles of handling interpersonal conflict. *Academy of Management Journal.* 1983;26(2):368–76.

39. Davis MH, Schoenfeld MB, Flores EJ. Predicting conflict acts using behavior and style measures. *International Journal of Conflict Management.* 2018;29(1):70–90.

40. Cherry MG, Fletcher I, O'Sullivan H, Dornan T. Emotional intelligence in medical education: A critical review. *Medical Education.* 2014;48(5):468–78.

41. Burke A. Group work: How to use groups effectively. *Journal of Effective Teaching.* 2011;11(2):87–95.

42. McKeachie W, Svinicki M. *McKeachie's Teaching Tips.* Cengage Learning; 2013.

43. Grasha AF, Yangarber-Hicks N. Integrating teaching styles and learning styles with instructional technology. *College Teaching.* 2000;48(1):2–10.

44. Bernstein S, Atkinson AR, Martimianakis MA. Diagnosing the learner in difficulty. *Pediatrics.* 2013;132(2):210–12.

45. Frei E, Stamm M, Buddeberg-Fischer B. Mentoring programs for medical students-a review of the PubMed literature 2000–2008. *BMC Medical Education.* 2010;10(1):32.

46. Moir F, Henning MA, Hassed C, Moyes SA, Elley CR. Peer program for mental health of medical students. *Teaching and Learning in Medicine.* 2016;28(3):293–302.

47. Souba WW. Mentoring young academic surgeons, our most precious asset. *Journal of Surgical Research.* 1999;82(2):113–20.

48. Hur Y. Development of a career coaching model for medical students. *Korean Journal of Medical Education.* 2016;28(1):127.

49. Kilminster S, Jolly B. Effective supervision in clinical practice settings: A literature review. *Medical Education.* 2000;34(10):827–40.

50. Nottingham S, Henning J. Feedback in clinical education, part I: Characteristics of feedback provided by approved clinical instructors. *Journal of Athletic Training.* 2014;49(1):49–57.

51. Kornegay JG, Kraut A, Manthey D, Omron R, Caretta-Weyer H, Kuhn G, et al. Feedback in medical education: A critical appraisal. *AEM Education and Training.* 2017;1(2):98–109.

52. Cantillon P, Sargeant J. Giving feedback in clinical settings. *BMJ.* 2008;337:a1961.

53. Tan CH, Lee SS, Yeo SP, Ashokka B, Samarasekera DD. Developing metacognition through effective feedback. *Medical Teacher.* 2016;38(9):959–62.

54. Telio S, Ajjawi R, Regehr G. The "educational alliance" as a framework for reconceptualizing feedback in medical education. *Academic Medicine.* 2015;90(5):609–14.

55. Arnold L, Shue CK, Kritt B, Ginsburg S, Stern DT. Medical students' views on peer assessment of professionalism. *Journal of General Internal Medicine.* 2005;20(9):819–24.

56. Sandars J. The use of reflection in medical education: AMEE Guide No. 44. *Medical Teacher.* 2009;31(8):685–95.

57. Kolb AY, Kolb DA. Learning styles and learning spaces: Enhancing experiential learning in higher education. *Academy of Management Learning & Education.* 2005;4(2):193–212.

58. Gibbs G. *Learning by Doing: A Guide to Teaching and Learning Methods.* Oxford: Further Education Unit, Oxford Brookes University; 1988.

59. Gaughf NW, Foster PS, Williams DA. Student-reported satisfaction with academic enhancement services at an academic health science center. *Education for Health.* 2014;27(2):208.

60. Murad MH, Varkey P. Self-directed learning in health professions education. *Annals Academy of Medicine Singapore.* 2008;37(7):580.

61. Puertas EB, Arósquipa C, Gutiérrez D. Factors that influence a career choice in primary care among medical students from high-, middle-, and low-income countries: A systematic review. *Revista Panamericana de Salud Pública.* 2013;34:351–8.

62. Pangerčić A, Sambunjak D, Hren D, Marušić M, Marušić A. Climate for career choices: Survey of medical students' motivation for studying, career preferences and perception of their teachers as role models. *Wiener Klinische Wochenschrift.* 2010;122(7–8):243–50.

63. Henning MA, Krägeloh C, Moir F, Hawken SJ, Lyndon MP, Hill AG. The quality of life of medical students and clinicians. In: Giardino AP, Giardino ER, editors. *Medical Education: Global Perspectives, Challenges and Future Directions.* New York: Nova Science Publishers, Inc.; 2013:231–50.

64. Sawir E, Marginson S, Deumert A, Nyland C, Ramia G. Loneliness and international students: An Australian study. *Journal of Studies in International Education.* 2008;12(2):148–80.

65. Moir F, Fernando III AT, Kumar S, Henning MA, Moyes SA, Elley CR. Computer Assisted Learning for the Mind (CALM): The mental health of medical students and their use of a self-help website. *New Zealand Medical Journal.* 2015;128(1411):51–58.

66. The University of Auckland. CALM — Computer Assisted Learning for the Mind; n.d. Available from: https://www.calm.auckland.ac.nz/index.html.

67. McFall RM, Townsend JT. Foundations of psychological assessment: Implications for cognitive assessment in clinical science. *Psychological Assessment.* 1998;10(4):316.

68. University of Tasmania. University behaviour policy; 2019. Available from: https://secure.utas.edu.au/__data/assets/pdf_file/0006/1181985/University-Behaviour-Policy.pdf.

69. University of Alberta. Code of student behaviour; 2018. Available from: https://www.ualberta.ca/governance/media-library/documents/resources/policies-standards-and-codes-of-conduct/cosb-updated-july-1-2019.pdf

70. Duke University School of Medicine. Code of professional conduct; 2017. Available from: https://medschool.duke.edu/sites/medschool.duke.edu/files/field/attachments/Code_of_Professional_Conduct.pdf.

71. Frellsen SL, Baker EA, Papp KK, Durning SJ. Medical school policies regarding struggling medical students during the internal medicine clerkships: Results of a national survey. *Academic Medicine.* 2008;83(9):876–81.

72. Lizzio A, Wilson K, Hadaway V. University students' perceptions of a fair learning environment: A social justice perspective. *Assessment & Evaluation in Higher Education.* 2007;32(2):195–213.

73. Green EP, Gruppuso PA. Justice and care: Decision making by medical school student promotions committees. *Medical Education*. 2017;51(6):621–32.

74. Colbert CY, French JC, Herring ME, Dannefer EF. Fairness: The hidden challenge for competency-based postgraduate medical education programs. *Perspectives on Medical Education*. 2017;6(5):347–55.

75. Ayala EE, Omorodion AM, Nmecha D, Winseman JS, Mason HR. What do medical students do for self-care? A student-centered approach to well-being. *Teaching and Learning in Medicine*. 2017;29(3):237–46.

76. Pellegrino ED. Professionalism, profession and the virtues of the good physician. *Mount Sinai Journal of Medicine*. 2002;69(6):378–84.

77. Askitopoulou H, Vgontzas AN. The relevance of the Hippocratic Oath to the ethical and moral values of contemporary medicine. Part I: The Hippocratic Oath from antiquity to modern times. *European Spine Journal*. 2018;27(7):1481–90.

78. Semradova I, Hubackova S. Responsibilities and competences of a university teacher. *Procedia-Social and Behavioral Sciences*. 2014;159:437–41.

79. Blaskova M, Blasko R, Matuska E, Rosak-Szyrocka J. Development of key competences of university teachers and managers. *Procedia-Social and Behavioral Sciences*. 2015;182:187–96.

80. The University of Auckland. Bachelor of Medicine and Bachelor of Surgery; 2019. Available from: https://www.auckland.ac.nz/en/study/study-options/find-a-study-option/bachelor-of-medicine-and-bachelor-of-surgery-mbchb.html.

81. Vázquez JL, Aza CL, Lanero A. Responsible human resources management in the university: A view of Spanish students. *Human Resources Management & Ergonomics*. 2014;8(1):118–28.

82. Steinert Y, Mann K, Centeno A, Dolmans D, Spencer J, Gelula M, et al. A systematic review of faculty development initiatives designed to improve teaching effectiveness in medical education: BEME Guide No. 8. *Medical Teacher*. 2006;28(6):497–526.

83. Sheehan DC. Learning and supervision in internship: A sociocultural framework for understanding learning and supervision in medical internship; 2010.

84. Koskina A. What does the student psychological contract mean? Evidence from a UK business school. *Studies in Higher Education*. 2013;38(7):1020–36.

85. Svensson G, Wood G. Are university students really customers? When illusion may lead to delusion for all! *International Journal of Educational Management*. 2007;21(1):17–28.

86. Appleton-Knapp SL, Krentler KA. Measuring student expectations and their effects on satisfaction: The importance of managing student expectations. *Journal of Marketing Education*. 2006;28(3):254–64.

87. Boehler ML, Rogers DA, Schwind CJ, Mayforth R, Quin J, Williams RG, et al. An investigation of medical student reactions to feedback: A randomised controlled trial. *Medical Education*. 2006;40(8):746–49.

88. Li S-TT, Paterniti DA, West DC. Successful self-directed lifelong learning in medicine: A conceptual model derived from qualitative analysis of a national survey of pediatric residents. *Academic Medicine*. 2010;85(7):1229–36.

LEADERSHIP AND MANAGEMENT IN MEDICAL AND HEALTH PROFESSIONS' EDUCATION: WHY DO I NEED TO LEAD?

Judy McKimm, Kirsty Forrest, Paul Jones, Tang Ching Lau

Scenario

Over the years, Dr Gina has become an excellent teacher, well liked by both her peers and students. As a senior clinician, she first started teaching students in practice and was appointed as a teacher in the School 14 years ago. Since then, she has been involved in many initiatives, twice won an award for her teaching and recently led a successful review of the undergraduate nursing curriculum. In the light of her many contributions to the School, 6 months ago she was appointed as the Dean of Learning and Teaching, responsible for the oversight and development of the School's undergraduate and postgraduate medical and health professions' programmes.

Dr Gina had been offered and had taken the role, despite having no formal qualifications in learning and teaching or educational management, as it was felt she was ready for the next stage of her career and that she could really make a difference to health professions' education in the School. However, she is finding the additional role overwhelming. Her relationship with her peers seems to have changed overnight; there is so much paperwork; she feels she hardly sees students and feels out of her depth in high-level university meetings where everyone else is so confident and knowledgeable. She is finding it increasingly challenging to prioritise and manage her workload and roll out new initiatives, including the new nursing programme, which she really enjoyed developing. She is not finding as much enjoyment in her job as before and is at a loss as to what she could do about the situation in which she finds herself.

She happens to be talking with a colleague one morning and explaining how she is feeling. Her colleague suggests that she attend a short leadership course, which is happening in a week or two. He suggests that this might help her learn more about what is expected of her and give her some ideas about next steps.

Introduction

In this section, we explore leadership and management in medical and health professions' education using a typical situation in which many people have found themselves: taking on a leadership role without much preparation.

What is happening to Dr Gina is very common, not only in universities and health professions' education, but in many organisations around the world. Widespread evidence exists that leadership and management are key to organisational success and efficiency, particularly in the VUCA (Volatile, Uncertain, Complex, Ambiguous) world in which we live.[1,2] Effective leadership promotes a positive culture and climate, and is central to the student learning experience, quality and improvement, but targeted leadership development and purposeful succession planning is typically either patchy or non-existent. Most of us are not 'born' into leadership, and we are certainly not born into leadership or management positions. We therefore need training on the requirements of the role, and professional development geared specifically around leadership and management. However, although there is much more recognition that leadership and management development is required for those in leadership positions, this is often either offered only when someone is in a leadership post or not at all.

Chapters 1–3 consider various aspects of leadership and management and what this means in practice. Chapter 1 defines leadership and its components and then considers various factors that help explain how and why Dr Gina has found herself in this situation. We next look at the skills and qualities that leaders working in health professions' education need, drawing on research from within medical and health professions' education as well as the wider leadership literature. Finally, we take a number of typical situations that health professions' education leaders have to deal with and offer practical strategies for coping with these.

Chapter 1: Why? — Why Does This Happen?

Before we start to discuss why situations like this happen and what can be done about it, it is helpful to define what we mean by leadership. The leadership course Dr Gina attended provides some of the theory and breaks it down into different aspects.

A model we have developed takes the ever-growing literature on leadership and condenses this into sets of 'threes', the 'petals' of a daffodil, see Figure 1. The 'Swansea daffodil' is based on the national flower of Wales, reflecting the Canadian CanMEDS 'daisy' framework, which describes the roles and competencies of a doctor.[3] Each of the three elements in the daffodil

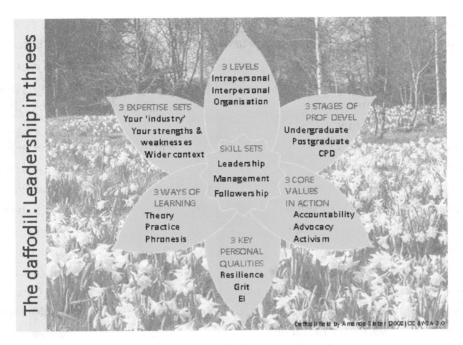

Fig. 1.   The Swansea daffodil: Leadership in threes.

petals summarise key aspects of leadership that have been identified from the literature and in practice. In the centre are the three core skill sets of **leadership, management and followership** that educational and clinical leaders need, we have called this the 'leadership triad' as it comprises the three interwoven components that are needed to be and become an effective leader.[4]

Thinking of the activities of a leader in terms of this triad is much more helpful and realistic than thinking that all 'managers' do is 'manage' and all that 'leaders' do is 'lead', because in practice everyone carries out some management and some leadership activities within their roles.

Organisations, teams and situations need both leadership and management in varying amounts depending on the context. Management is about efficiency, planning, providing stability and order, whereas leadership is about effectiveness, change, setting direction and adaptability. Drucker[5] suggests that organisations need both a management perspective, including 'doing things right' (efficiency) coupled with the leadership perspective of 'doing the right things' (effectiveness). He makes the point that it is no use being highly efficient if you are doing the wrong things. For example, a health professions' programme might be managed very well and run like clockwork, but if it is out of date and does not meet regulatory standards, then educational leadership is needed to create a vision for the right change needed, and both leadership and management are required to ensure the vision for a new programme turns into reality. Mowbray[6] makes a helpful distinction in noting that 'processes need managers and management, people need leaders and leadership' (p. 2). So, in our health professions' programme example, whilst it is important to ensure that the new programme is mapped to the professional standards, that the timetable activities are achievable and that assessments can be managed with existing resources (management activities), it is the people involved who will make the programme come to life, and motivate and nurture the health professionals of tomorrow, and that requires good leadership.

Finally, we do not lead all the time, however senior we are in an organisation or profession. There are always people who are more expert or better at certain things than we are ourselves, so being able to be a good 'follower' (who is supportive, active, questioning and helpful) is vital to ensure groups, teams and organisations function smoothly. And leaders need to be able to communicate with and motivate their own 'followers', both team members and those who they influence more widely. Denhardt and Denhardt talk about leadership being an art (a 'dance'), which involves fluidity, rhythm, passion, expression, improvisation, interpretation, focus, discipline and an awareness of space, time and energy.[7] We also like to think of this 'dance of leadership' as involving a deft, seamless stepping in and out, forward and back, between leadership, management and followership. So, we see part of the art of leadership as about knowing when and how to manage well, when to follow, and when you or others need to step up and take leadership.

Definitions and Theories of Leadership, Management and Followership

Having said that it is essential that leaders (and managers) can perform a mix of different activities, the well-established literature often distinguishes between leadership and management, with followership having a much more recent history. More recently, leadership theorists are thinking (as discussed above) that whilst there are distinctions between leadership and management activities, it is the continued interplay of these activities by and within individuals and teams that makes organisations most effective. Leadership, management and followership are all social constructs, they are shaped by sociocultural influences and the zeitgeist of the time, and are constantly being mediated, reshaped and reconstructed.

Leadership

Kurt Lewin said that 'there is nothing as practical as a good theory', and in this section, we select some of the most relevant leadership theories (from the many that exist) and explain their real-world practical application to practise in health professions' education.[8] Many writers (including ourselves) have written about leadership theories, and the literature is vast, so here we provide a summary of theories, a framework for thinking about them, and refer

Table 1.   Major leadership theories and concepts.

Adaptive, complex adaptive leadership	Implicit leadership theories (ILTs)
Affective leadership	Inclusive leadership
Authentic leadership	Leader–member exchange (LMX) theory
Charismatic leadership, narcissistic	Ontological leadership
Collaborative, collective, shared leadership	Person-centred leadership
Contingency theories	Phenomenological leadership
Destructive, toxic (the dark triad) leadership	Relational leadership
Dialogic leadership	Servant leadership
Distributed, dispersed (shared) leadership	Situational leadership
Eco leadership	Spiritual leadership
Emotional Intelligence (EI)	Trait theory, 'great man' theory
Engaging leadership	Transactional leadership
Expert leadership	Transformational leadership
Followership	Value-led, moral leadership

Key: Red — primarily intrapersonal; Purple — primarily interpersonal; Green — organisation or system

to others throughout the section where relevant. Table 1 sets out some of the major theories and approaches, and you may well have already heard of some of the more common ones, such as Situational Leadership, Transformational Leadership and Emotional Intelligence (EI). Some of these theories have been criticised for being 'leader-centric', seeing the leader as the focus in terms of their influence, power and control, rather than the interplay between followers and leaders, but they remain very dominant.

As set out in the Daffodil model, we find it helpful for people to make sense of the theories and apply them to their own development and situation by categorising them broadly into three levels, although some theories fall into more than one. These are described below, in broad chronological order, and it should be noted that, as in education, new theories do not replace former ones, but our thinking about leadership is reframed as we look through different 'lenses'. So, theories that have been very influential in the past still continue to frame our thinking about leadership today.

1. *Understanding yourself as a leader*

These theories focus on the personal qualities or personality of the leader as an individual and help us get to know ourselves better, develop self-insight into why we do things a certain way, understand our strengths and weaknesses, and how we respond under pressure.

Early theories of leadership focussed on the 'great man' or 'heroic leader', one (usually a man) who was authoritative and acted as a figurehead for their organisation, cause or country. These people became leaders by virtue of their position in society, sometimes this was bestowed upon them through heredity (e.g. monarchy) although more often it was based on their actual and perceived skills, qualities and abilities as a leader (e.g. in industry or government, religion, the military). Whilst cultural variations exist, certain personality traits, personal qualities and behaviours were subsequently seen as more 'leaderful' than others. The qualities ascribed to leaders therefore arose from a combination of factors (see Table 2).

These traditional views persist today, although they have been tempered by more recent theories and concepts, some of which challenge these traditional views, others which complement them. A key shift was that, from the 1960s onwards, many writers started to challenge the idea that leaders and managers were born (to certain positions, or with certain characteristics) and began to highlight not only that different leadership styles or approaches could be adopted, contingent on different situations or contexts, but also that leadership could be 'learned'.[9-11] Underpinning this shift were developments in the social and behavioural sciences, which started to see personality traits and identity as not necessarily fixed from birth or early childhood, but which could be modified and adapted throughout life. More recent literature focuses on this growth and development through life, for example, Nonaka and Takeuchi's concept of the 'wise leader' emphasises that a leader[12]:

- Needs more than knowledge alone
- Can practise moral discernment
- Can sum up complex situations quickly and grasp key essence of problems
- Creates the context for organisational learning
- Communicates effectively
- Exercises political power judiciously
- Fosters development of practical wisdom in others

The wise leader therefore needs to have developed their own 'practical wisdom' (phronesis), which can only be achieved through experience, reflection and personal growth. The Japanese concept of Ikigai (meaning 'reason for being'),[13,14] Sinek's[15] work on finding your 'why' (your core purpose) and Duckworth's concept of 'grit',[16] also see leadership as being centred within a person's whole life, involving combinations of passion, core purpose, resilience, direction, perseverance, values, achievement and self-worth. Recent leadership research in this area, drawing from linguistics, philosophy and psychology, moves away from what a leader 'does' to who they 'are': the 'being and becoming' a leader (ontology). This includes work on leader identity formation; notions of power, authority and control[17]; dominant leadership discourses, and ontological

Table 2. Traditional perspectives of leadership and their impact on our understanding.

How traditional perspectives on leaders and leadership emerged	Impact on our understanding of leadership and leaders
Sociocultural beliefs about the place of certain groups and individuals in society, which vary between cultures and over time, including: • Social stratification, e.g. social class, caste systems, where some are at the 'top' (leaders) and the rest are at the 'bottom' (followers) • That women's place is 'at home' and men are 'breadwinners' • That leadership relates to the world of 'work' • A belief that leaders were somehow 'born' not 'made'	This varies between cultures and over time, but in general has led to some individuals and groups believing and acting as they were destined for leadership, others that they could never become leaders
Symbolism around leadership and leaders	Throughout history, in art (paintings and sculptures), speech and theatre, leaders have been portrayed as and celebrated for being 'larger than life', 'heroic' and 'godlike'. Such symbolism around leaders and their powers is highly pervasive and leads to the belief that leadership is all about seniority, power and 'big L' leadership
Legacies from tribal times, including social and neurobiological influences	Certain personality and physical traits and qualities became associated with leaders, e.g. height, strength, 'perfection', charisma, confidence and good communication skills
Who leaders actually were at various times in history — the visible leaders were not necessarily representative of the whole population	Because the visible 'great' leaders were men, typically high-born or seen as having leadership bestowed upon them by a higher power, people who did not fit these characteristics could not be leaders

leadership. For example, Souba[18] suggests that four ontological pillars underpin the 'being' of leadership: awareness, commitment, integrity and authenticity, whereas McKenna and Rooney[19] focus on leaders developing 'ontological acuity', being aware of organisational knowledge systems and discourses.

In health professions' education, our work is predominantly 'people work', involving emotional labour with learners and faculty, requiring 'affective leadership' (building strong emotional connections and relationships) and therefore a highly controlling 'hero leader' approach is often counter-productive. The idea of 'Servant leadership', a concept first coined by Greenleaf, has gained traction in recent years with its strong connection to values and public service. Core personal principles in servant leadership such as to wanting to serve first and make a difference to people's lives; take a facilitative approach; focus on caring, well-being and healing, and stewardship (taking care of something that is not yours, improving it and handing it on to your successor) are very relevant to education and healthcare.[20] Value-based and moral leadership are also closely linked to servant leadership, where the leader takes a moral stance, whose values are transparent and which underpin their behaviours and actions. Whilst the 'expert' leader is highly prized for their leadership around their specific expertise, we cannot be an expert in everything, so learning to listen and value those around you for their strengths and expertise is vital in our context. Theories, which focus on an individual's EI, authenticity and values as core leadership strengths help explain why some leadership approaches 'work' and others do not. Seeing these leadership qualities as strengths allow us to accept leaders who are imperfect, human and who make mistakes — fallible leaders — as long as these leaders have the EI to recognise this, listen to others and change.

2. *Leading and working with others*

These theories relate to the way in which a leader interacts with others. They help us work in and lead teams, and communicate with and influence others more effectively. The influential shift towards thinking that leaders and leadership could be developed led to a wide range of general literature, research and development activities aiming to identify the issues that aspiring and existing leaders needed to address to become 'successful'.

For many years, the focus was on developing the individual leader's skills and understanding, with the leader being seen as the most powerful and influential actor in encounters. We call these 'leader-centric' approaches. Some of these have been discussed above, such as developing higher social or emotional intelligence and adopting the 'right' leadership style or approach for different contexts or situations. Other theories or concepts, prominent in the health and education contexts, focus on the leader's role in leading change through and with people, the importance of building and sustaining relationships, and the generation of positive dialogues and discourses. Transformational leadership, for example, is grounded in humanistic psychology and is about leaders inspiring and motivating others towards higher order goals or values. Bass[21] talks about the 'four I's' of transformational leadership:

- Idealised influence — involves the leader influencing through acting as a good role model
- Inspirational motivation — motivating others through inspiring them to better things

- Intellectual stimulation — motivating people by stimulating them intellectually
- Individualised consideration — paying attention to the needs and aspirations of individual team members

This contrasts with transactional leadership which involves exchange of effort for reward (e.g. you work for an employer and you get paid). Of course, many work encounters are transactional, but the approaches in which leaders achieve meaningful change whilst also developing people have been highly influential, despite the difficulty of being truly 'transformational' within the midst of austerity, managed systems, targets and performance measures.

More recently however (see below) more attention is being paid to the interaction of leaders and 'followers', acknowledging that such interactions are part of complex dynamic processes, not linear or one-way. Reflecting this, approaches that embody the belief that leadership needs to be a collective process in which people are central have emerged. Such approaches include distributed, shared, collective and collaborative leadership. These approaches are different, but have common features:

- Leadership is seen as a process: teamwork and co-creation is important, only by working together will improvement be made
- Power shared gives more power for all to use
- Rather than focussing just on individual leader development, building social capital and leadership capacity throughout the organisation is essential — leadership and expertise is distributed at all levels
- Leadership is emergent and boundaries are open so that knowledge and learning is shared

Two relatively recent approaches which seem very relevant to health professions' education are 'person-centred' leadership and 'inclusive leadership'.[22,23] Person-centred leadership involves operating from your strengths and allowing others to compensate for your limitations, encouraging others around you, and building a culture around a shared vision by knowing and sharing why you do what you do.[15] Inclusive leaders build relationships with others that can accomplish things for mutual benefit; do things with people rather than to people — the essence of inclusion; values, promotes and encourages diversity; and actively addresses unconscious and implicit biases through training, development and challenging inappropriate behaviours. Both these approaches emphasise organisational empathy; valuing people for who they are, as well as for what they do; they take a moral stance, and incorporate values-based leadership. Finally, 'caring',[24] 'courageous'[15] and 'compassionate' leadership[25,26] have been applied to healthcare and other settings; again these approaches would seem to be the sort of leadership we might strive towards in our context.

3. *Leadership in organisations or systems*

This group of theories seek to explain leadership behaviours in relation to the environment or system, much of which draws from management and organisational psychology literature. They guide us in learning about and understanding the wider systems and organisations in which we work, understanding politics and processes, and determining strategies for managing and leading change and improvement initiatives. As mentioned, servant, value-based and moral leadership are all very relevant approaches, involving 'making a difference' through engaging with the moral purpose and values of an organisation. The recent concept of 'eco-leadership' builds on these approaches, emphasising the concepts of stewardship, and environmental, societal and organisational sustainability.[27] This is crucial for healthcare and education, echoing the United Nations' seventeen Sustainable Development Goals, developed to address global challenges faced by the international community, including poverty, inequality, climate, environmental degradation, prosperity and peace and justice, so that no one is left behind.[28,29]

It is becoming increasingly clear we are living in a VUCA (Volatile, Uncertain, Complex, Ambiguous) world, which requires leaders to have a growth mindset, and organisations, which are flexible enough (in their structures, people and organisations) to adapt to changing conditions.[2,30] The most effective leaders have therefore learned to understand and navigate organisations and systems; they are boundary-spanners; they can take a systems-thinking approach and are flexible, adapting to both internal and external change drivers. 'Adaptive leadership' describes leaders who are comfortable working in complex, uncertain systems and times and can adapt their ways of working to develop solutions to new or 'wicked' problems (problems with no clear solution).[31,32] Bolman and Gallos[33] suggest that one way academic leaders can do this is by looking through different lenses or 'frames' (the structural, human resource, political and symbolic frames) to provide different perspectives on their organisations and tackle issues in different ways.

Management

The practice and theories that underpin modern management have a long history. Management was first conceptualised in efficiency studies in the 16th century, further developed as industries and factories were introduced and refined as service industries became prominent. Management is primarily about planning and order, relating to the structures, co-ordination, organisation and administration of a business's activities to achieve its goals or objectives.

Management activities therefore include developing strategy and policy; controlling the means and processes of production; finances; innovation; and marketing and promotion. It involves managing resources, be they physical (buildings, equipment), human (people), natural (water, oxygen) or technological (computer, other systems).

Most organisations have three levels of management:

- Senior managers (e.g. the chief executive, president, finance director, etc.) who carry out the more strategic aspects, setting and planning a strategy and objectives, and who decide how the organisation will operate. They delegate and manage the next tier down.
- Middle managers who act as the interface and communication channel (sometimes the buffer) between the senior managers and the frontline managers. These would include department heads, programme directors or directors of administrative units.
- Lower managers, frontline managers or supervisors, such as heads of assessment, course or module leads. These oversee the work of others and often have a frontline aspect to their work, dealing directly with customers, students or patients.

In health professions' education, many individuals hold a number of roles and tasks, which overlap and cut across structural lines of responsibility and accountability. Swanwick and McKimm set out the key management skills which health professions' educators need to be able to do, which can be summarised as follows[34]:

- Understanding, controlling and managing budgets
- Human resource (people) management
- Physical resources and facilities
- Business planning (e.g. strategic, departmental and operational plans)
- Curriculum/programme management and timetabling
- Project management
- Understanding the internal environment
- Understanding the external environment
- Understanding and developing management systems (including IT) and processes
- Educational quality, evaluation
- Time management (self and others)
- Chairing or being involved in committees

For example, the assessment lead of an undergraduate course might be responsible for planning assessments and managing others to carry out the essential tasks, chairing meetings and producing examination papers. They might also lead on a module relating to their specific discipline and therefore attend curriculum or programme management meetings, as well as be an academic mentor for some first year students. In light of their assessment expertise they might also be part of a national body, again with different responsibilities, and also be the principal investigator for a multi-centre research study, holding a national grant.

We like to think of management as maintaining stability and order, enabling forward planning of resources and activities, and a means to monitor and evaluate successes and failings. In curriculum terms, the management required includes the strategic development of the programme, mapped against internal and external benchmarks and standards, and a realistic and feasible programme design in light of educational needs and available resources. For example, it is no good planning an intensive case, problem or inquiry-based course, which requires many small group teaching rooms and facilities, if these are not available or of insufficient quality. Curriculum mapping and assessment blueprinting are also essential management activities, which assure yourselves and the regulators that learning outcomes are taught, learned and assessed appropriately. Whilst these activities will require some leadership, they also require management skills, which can be learned over time.[35]

As you can see, there is no point having a great vision and ideas if these cannot be translated into reality that works on the ground. Indeed, Gosling and Mintzberg go further, saying that '*the separation of management from leadership is dangerous. Just as management without leadership encourages an uninspired style, which deadens activities, leadership without management encourages a disconnected style, which promotes hubris. And we all know the destructive power of hubris in organisations*'[36] (p.1). So, management and leadership skills are both needed for objectives to be met, but in various amounts by different people in different contexts. Those with a formal designation of 'manager' will still lead people and tasks, and those with a leadership role need to be able to manage workflow and outputs.[37]

Followership

Followership is the most recent of the three concepts comprising the 'leadership triad'. For many writers, the focus on 'leadership' (the 'leader-centric approach') has led to a paucity of research into followers and followership. The predominance of the individualised concepts of leadership described above (e.g. the 'hero leader', 'great man', charismatic and transformational leadership) conceptualised followers either as subordinates, as passive recipients of and responders to leaders' actions, influence and instructions, or as constructors of what leaders and leadership mean.[38] As leadership became conceptualised in terms of a social construct and process, created and mediated through interaction and relationships between people, so followership is seen as essential, as without followers, there are no leaders.[38] The study of followership however, is relatively recent, with most studies having been carried out in the last 15 years.

Role-based approaches consider followership in terms of formal hierarchical roles (e.g. subordinate, deputy), 'seeing followers as causal agents and leaders as recipients or moderators of followership outcomes'[38] (p. 85). This perspective has contributed towards the term 'follower' having a negative connotation, which privileges and romanticises leadership and subordinates followership. The most recent writers therefore make a distinction between 'leaders' (who exert social influence over others) and 'followers' (who are willing to defer to and interact with others). From this perspective, the 'exemplary' or 'star' follower is an engaged and active agent, willing to collaborate in a common purpose, supporting their leaders yet speaking out when they think things are wrong.[39,40] Chaleff[41] suggests such followers are 'courageous' as they are willing to 'stand up to and for leaders' and are accountable for their actions.

Most of the research on followership sees followership behaviours either in terms of a relationship between deference and dominance (the follower 'agrees' to defer to or be influenced by the leader for various reasons) or, from a constructivist perspective, that the follower takes on a follower 'identity' and grants the leader a leader 'identity'.[42] Implicit followership theories (IFTs) suggest that, just as we hold implicit theories of leadership, which are socially constricted and mediated and often held unconsciously, so too do we hold unconscious but pervasive ideas about what, who, why and how we should follow some leaders, but not others. This often leads to a categorisation of leaders as either 'good' or 'bad'. Such judgements affect the way followers interact with various leaders, and how followers interact with one another. From a social identity perspective, this can lead to the development of collective emotion, including support for and movements against leaders or the development of in-groups and out-groups in which some followers feel that they belong, whereas others feel or are marginalised or excluded.[43,44]

Probably, most leaders try to do the best they can, given the circumstances and the teams in which they find themselves. However, some leaders are perceived by their followers as toxic or destructive because of their behaviours, actions and inactions. Some leaders are destructive because they are out of their depth or feel they have to do everything themselves. This can lead to followers feeling micro-managed, or alternatively abandoned. Leaders who are weak or who don't know what they are doing do not gain the respect of their followers and once trust is lost (e.g. through breaking promises, poor communication, ineptitude or lack of knowledge), it is virtually impossible to regain. Other leaders are toxic because of their personality traits or other variables. Such toxic leaders may display a lack of empathy and understanding of others' wants and needs; may be arrogant and self-serving; sabotage or take credit for others' work or achievements; may have favourites amongst the group; may bully and harass people or be unpredictable. The 'dark triad' of personalities describes three overlapping, offensive but non-pathological personalities: Machiavellianism, subclinical narcissism and subclinical psychopathy.[45] In leadership, this leads to interesting paradoxes for both leaders and followers:

- Leaders need to be (and appear to be) self-confident and have strong self-belief — but not appear arrogant, grandiose, entitled, superior or dominant, i.e. display narcissistic behaviours
- Leaders need to be seen as calm, be able to make tough (sometimes unpopular) decisions, appear strong (which may involve disciplining or firing people), and be able to take calculated risks — but not appear emotionally cold, lacking in empathy or anxiety, or show high impulsivity and thrill seeking i.e. display psychopathic behaviours
- Leaders need to be able to work the politics of the organisational 'jungle' and 'manage' people — but not be seen as manipulative, i.e. display Machiavelliansim

Leaders therefore need to be aware of how their behaviours might appear to others and where more person-centred and inclusive approaches can be used.

Summary

In this chapter, we take the three levels at which leadership operates: the intrapersonal, interpersonal and organisation or system level (identified in the 'Swansea daffodil') and explore some of the useful leadership, management and followership skills at each level, noting that some things do not fall easily into one level. We have looked at some of the theories underpinning leadership, management and followership and highlighted how these can help our understanding and started to use the Swansea 'Leadership in threes' daffodil to explore some of the various facets of educational leadership as they relate to Dr Gina's situation.

In Chapters 2 and 3, we look at the skills that leaders need and how to use these in practice at the three levels and explore the approaches, knowledge, skills and competencies leaders can use to both develop themselves and become an effective leader.

Practice Highlights

- Moving into a leadership role poses challenges and dilemmas as well as opportunities for growth and challenge
- The many theories and concepts of leadership that exist can help us develop as health professions' education leaders

- Our activities and development occurs at three levels: the intrapersonal, interpersonal and the organisation/system
- Leadership involves a combination of leadership activities, management tasks and being a follower

Chapter 2: What? — What Are The Useful Tools/Skills For A Leader?

Scenario

Dr Gina has had many thoughts after attending the leadership course. Moving into a more senior position, whether you want it or not, involves some customisation of our social identity as we adapt to being seen differently by others and having to develop 'leaderfulness'. This is challenging, and Dr Gina is displaying what is commonly termed 'imposter syndrome': she feels as if she an imposter in the Dean's role and that everyone else knows more and is more of an expert than she is. It is rather like the tale of 'the Emperor's new clothes', we feel under-equipped for or not worthy of the role, that everyone is just waiting for us to reveal that we are an imposter, and we will be found out. Dr Gina is also very conscious that she has no formal teaching or educational qualifications, which will exacerbate feeling like an imposter in the new role. Building credibility as a leader takes time and confidence, and whether Dr Gina is aware of it or not, she will have her own beliefs about what 'good' senior health professions' leaders do and don't, what they look like and what they don't. Internationally, women are under-represented at senior levels in a range of organisations, including universities. If there are few women role models in such jobs in the university, then it can be difficult if you 'don't fit the mould', feeling as if you have to prove yourself over and over again.

Dr Gina is struggling with feeling overwhelmed with the volume of work and rapidly finding out just what a heavy managerial and administrative burden these academic roles entail. Not only is she having to attend meetings, manage people and think more strategically, but she is also still working clinically, whereas often these roles are taken by academics who work full-time in the university. We call this the 'double burden' of health professions' leadership. What also happens when people move into new leadership positions or roles is that, because they are taking on new responsibilities, they usually need to give things up. All change therefore involves some type of loss as well as gain and, while a role transition is happening, this can be psychologically uncomfortable, particularly when the things we are 'losing' are the things that brought us into the job in the first place. For Dr Gina these were a love of students and teaching as well as curriculum development. Dr Gina is also in a transition period in which she will (almost inevitably, but hopefully temporarily) lose competence and confidence until she finds her feet in the new role.

Dr Gina knows the organisation and its culture well as she has worked there for many years, and this is an advantage. However, she has now moved up the hierarchy and has more organisational positional power and authority amongst her peers than she did before. Managing this shift can be difficult, as her colleagues (and students) may feel differently about her and will have to renegotiate their formal 'work' relationship. This can lead to feelings of isolation and, coupled with Gina feeling out of her depth, is probably contributing to her loss of enjoyment.

Dr Gina is encouraged by attending the leadership course and feels she understands more about leadership, what it is and what it isn't, and she is keen to learn more about some of the specific tools and skills that she will need in her new role.

Understanding Yourself: Your Strengths and Weaknesses

As part of the follow-up activities from her course, Dr Gina had completed a number of self-development activities on these topics and she felt that, although some of the results were a little confronting, her self-assessment of her strengths and areas for development was pretty accurate. One of the useful things she learned was the importance of having a positive approach to life, which, as a teacher and leader, is really important. Seligman's PERMA model comprises five core elements that underpin psychological well-being: Positive emotion (being optimistic about the past, present and future); Engagement (in activities that we enjoy and which absorbs us in the moment); Relationships (and strong social connections); Meaning (and finding purpose in our life and work) and Accomplishments (goals, ambitions and achievements).[46] From undertaking a series of self-development activities, she also learned that she had a 'growth mindset' rather than a 'fixed mindset' i.e. her view of the world is positive; setbacks are seen as temporary, not permanent; she has an underpinning belief that she can continue to learn and develop, and that effort will lead to achievement.[47] Table 3 has some more descriptions of characteristics of the different fixed and growth mindsets. Reflecting on how these concepts applied to her, Dr Gina realised that having a growth mindset and a good sense of psychological well-being had probably contributed to her achievements as a

Table 3.   Characteristics of fixed and growth mindsets.

Characteristic	Fixed mindset	Growth mindset
Skills/intelligence	I'm not good enough	What am I missing?
Goals	I need the outcome to be a success	I want to grow and learn
Feedback	I take feedback personally and get defensive	I like feedback and use it to learn
Challenges	If something is too hard, I give up	I keep trying even when I'm frustrated
Mistakes	It's not my fault — it was someone else's	Mistakes help me learn

clinician and teacher, and that she was operating successfully as a *'little "I"'* education leader already. She was starting to feel much more optimistic about her future role.[48]

Alongside these concepts which relate to the general population, the leadership literature identifies many personal qualities of effective leaders (e.g. integrity, humility and charisma) as well as the harmful effect of *toxic* or *destructive* leadership. However three qualities consistently emerge from studies of successful leaders: **resilience** — the ability to 'bounce back' from adversity or challenge[49]; **emotional intelligence** (EI) — a combination of self-awareness, empathy, social awareness, self-motivation and self-management[50,51]; and **'grit'** — a combination of resilience, passion, hard work, perseverance, determination and direction.[16] There is a lot of crossover between all these theories and concepts, with a sense of purpose, a positive mindset and a willingness to work hard being crucial to all. For example, Sinek talks about leaders finding their 'why', the core purpose that drives and motivates them, and a core aspect of maintaining resilience is being able to draw from spirituality, your beliefs, values and sense of purpose.[15]

Writers are still debating the extent to which these are types of personality traits or cognitive functions. For example, EI has been described in two different (but not mutually exclusive) ways. Salovey and Mayer[52] define 'ability EI' as the cognitive ability to monitor one's own and others' feelings and emotions, and to use this information to guide thinking and actions, whereas Petrides et al.[53] describe 'trait EI' as involving emotion-rated self-perceptions, similar to a personality trait of self-efficacy. However, whilst some people may appear more 'naturally' resilient, emotionally intelligent or 'gritty', research on neuroplasticity suggests that these can all be developed further, once people become aware of what they need to do and apply themselves to such learning.[54] We suggest that it is helpful to think of this as an integrated developmental process (*three A's*) in which leaders learn to develop *awareness* of their emotions and feelings, identifying what is happening both in their heads (e.g. feeling angry) and their bodies (e.g. clenching fists, increased heart rate); *accepting* that they are feeling such emotions; and then deciding (using rational cognition) what (if anything) to do about it (*action*).

Building Credibility

Some of the main things that followers want from their leader are to be valued, acknowledged and praised, and for their potential to be spotted, nurtured and developed: in other words, to be emotionally intelligent. And an inclusive, person-centred leader involves their followers in activities, allowing them to compensate for their weaknesses. However, before a leader can do this, they need to feel self-confident, it is hard to admit weakness or fallibility when you are unsure of yourself. Another aspect to this is that, influenced by implicit leadership theories, both followers and leaders may expect leaders to demonstrate certain characteristics: such as being strong, expert, authoritative and outgoing. So from a followership perspective, this is all about being credible as a leader as without this, followers simply won't follow you. Through our work with developing doctors-in-training in leadership, we suggest three expertise sets can help build your credibility.[55] These are at the top left of the Daffodil model.

First, by understanding your **'industry'** (e.g. healthcare education):

- know how healthcare and education systems, structures, funding and programmes work
- possess clinical and educational knowledge, so you can speak the languages (medical and education jargon)
- understand the wider sociocultural, political and economic context, to keep abreast of trends and policies

Secondly, becoming an **'expert'** in your area, project or initiative helps to build credibility, particularly when your power and influence is relatively low because of position in the organisation and professional hierarchies. Although Dr Gina feels she lacks an educational qualification, she has good experience of the curriculum review process in the university and is a highly experienced teacher, so this is what she needs to draw on. It could be that Dr Gina decides that having a formal qualification in education will give her more credibility (particularly in terms of learning theories), but in practice that might not be needed as she already knows a lot and could read around relevant subjects.

Finally (as with all professional roles), understanding your **strengths and weaknesses** helps you to build and work in effective teams and structure your leadership development.

Communications and Conversations

Many of the skills and approaches discussed above relate to the leader's interaction with others and communication skills. For example a core component of EI involves relationship building and managing which includes influencing skills; coaching and mentoring; teamwork; conflict management and inspirational leadership.[51] In order to effect change, motivate and inspire others, leaders need to be able to influence others, by expressing themselves clearly in different situations and contexts. Influencing involves a combination of advocacy, persuasion and negotiation, adapting your approach and style so that what you are saying appeals to others, engages them and helps build relationships. Some people will appreciate a rational style, with facts and figures, some will be influenced by your values, others will need a combination of approaches. Learning as much as you can about your team and the people you need to influence is vital, so that you can get people on your side or persuade them to your way of thinking.

Of course, not all communications are straightforward and this is where having self-insight is also important, so that you can recognise your effect on others. In Chapter 1, we looked at the traits and behaviours of 'toxic' leaders and mentioned the 'dark triad'. Understanding the impact of potentially destructive behaviours on others (such as undermining, not trusting, playing people off against each other or micro-managing) is helpful so we can try to avoid this. Recently, researchers have identified what they call the 'light triad' of personality.[56] Like the 'dark triad', this also involves three dimensions: Humanism (valuing the dignity and worth of each individual); Faith in humanity (believing in the fundamental goodness of humans) and Kantianism (treating people as ends unto themselves, not as mere means to an end). Aspects of the light triad fit well with some leadership approaches, with the healthcare and education contexts, and with what learners and colleagues expect from us. For example, Kouzes and Posner[57] talk about leaders making an inner journey in which they learn about themselves and what they care about, with this knowledge they can then lead and encourage other from their 'heart' and with kindness. This reflected in the healthcare leadership literature in terms of 'caring'[2,26] and 'compassionate' leadership.[25] So, a leader must be able to articulate their own values clearly, relate these both to the organisation's and team's needs and goals, and demonstrate that they do care about people through purposeful and intentional behaviours and actions: person-centred leadership.

Leading and working with others in teams and groups is probably where most of a leader's energy and time is expended, and this is essential for team formation and bonding, and for being able to delegate with confidence. The early literature on team-working focussed on group dynamics and the leader's role in facilitating effective group formation and working (e.g. Tuckman's theory of the stages groups go through 'forming'; "storming', norming', 'performing').[58]

This was complemented by a focus on team roles, which suggested that effective teams needed members to take a combination of roles, which can be divided into *People-oriented* roles (which consider group harmony and the needs of team members), *Action-oriented* roles (which focus on making things happen and achieving goals) and *Thinking-oriented* roles (which bring ideas and expertise to the team).[59]

Culture

'Culture is a set of living relationships working towards a shared goal'.[60]

The influence of leaders on culture has had increasing emphasis in literature and especially in the new generation of leadership theories. Thinking explicitly and working on culture will help a leader be more effective. In a recent book, *The Culture Code*, Daniel Coyle looked at highly successful teams across all industries from sport, the defence forces and hospitals to find out what they had in common. From his research he identified three skills that leaders had to emphasise to build a successful team:[60]

1. *Build safety for everyone to feel comfortable in working together*

Belonging needs to be continually refreshed and reinforced. Building safety includes listening (really listening), creating safe places where every one's voice is heard, valuing people and giving them a sense of belonging. Often a leader inherits a team which has history and relationships that may have broken down in the past, and where they have been 'led' autocratically and with punishment when things didn't go well. It can be particularly hard to establish psychological safety in such a scenario, and the first step is recognising that the team is not dysfunctional, they just don't trust the leader or the process. Practical steps a leader can take include: asking in one-to-one meetings 'What is one thing that I currently do that you would like me to continue to do?' and 'What is one thing that I don't do frequently enough that I should do more often?'. Leaders need to create safe spaces for working together, where everyone is heard, and allow people to have fun at work as well as being serious.

2. *Share vulnerability to show no one needs to be (or is) perfect*

Embrace failure as learning, many assume that to show vulnerability one would have to establish trust first. However, research suggests that showing and sharing vulnerability leads to trust and has been described as a vulnerability loop leading to contagious cooperation. Many of these aspects align with Brené Browns research on leadership, which highlights courage and vulnerability.[61] Her TED talk[62] has been viewed by over 35 million viewers. She emphasises having courageous conversations and leaning into vulnerability in her book 'Dare to Lead'.[63] Much of this is about accepting the emotion and uncomfortableness that one can feel in certain situations. She describes how that unease lasts on average 8 seconds, whereas when you do not have the discourse needed, the unease can last for weeks! The sharing of vulnerability must start with the leader, for example, acknowledging when they have made a mistake, asking if anybody has any ideas to help them and explicitly sharing the risk. Some organisations have a 'failure wall', where people reveal their failures, reflecting vulnerability and sharing learning.

3. *Establish purpose through a common goal and a clear path to get there*

Overcommunicate priorities. As a team, you are working in the 'now' towards a future common goal. The goal must be articulated, and the picture painted about how everyone is going to get there. Naming and ranking your top priorities is important, as well as identifying the team roles in achieving them. Catch phrases are helpful for explaining your values and can become common parlance, one of this chapter authors uses *'sprinkling kindness like confetti'* to espouse the value of kindness, which has been adopted by their team.

These three skills, which leaders would develop in a successful team, can be summarised as 'we are safe, we share risk and we know what it is all for.'

Culture and Conflict

Leaders need to promote a culture in which cognitive diversity and inclusivity is valued, but that this should not be too 'nice' a culture in which *'challenge, debate and heated discussion with a range of voices and opinions are not common for fear of upsetting the niceness balance and a desire to remain comfortable'.*[64] Conflict can occur when people have different perspectives or beliefs (they disagree), they misunderstand a situation or they have a different understanding of it (they see it differently). Some conflict is task-related (cognitive or substantive) involving different views on how to make a work-based decision or carry out an activity, others are affective (interpersonal or relationship-based) characterised by interpersonal negative emotions, such as anger or frustration. Of course tasks involve people working together, but poor relationships can undermine teams and activities. A key aspect of building and sustaining teams is therefore to develop trustful, safe relationships, not only so that teams can work productively but also have a space where 'fierce conversations' can be held and where substantive conflicts can be resolved. Interpersonal conflicts should be managed outside the team structure. Leaders need to be able to 'manage' and defuse conflict situations when they become unhelpful and The King's Fund suggests seven strategies[64]:

- 'Cultivate a growth mindset
- Welcome conflict as healthy
- Create psychological safety
- Encourage cognitive diversity

- Get comfortable with emotion
- Make development central to everyone's job
- Focus on creating a culture of dignity and respect for all'

Leaders also need to be aware of the sources of their power. 'Power' is often seen in a negative light and of course abuse of power is harmful, but we think it is more helpful to think of power in terms of where leaders draw their energy from. Raven suggests that there are six bases of social power we can draw from in different situations: expertise, reward, coercion, legitimacy, reference and information.[65] In a 'nasty' culture, power is overtly used to shut conflict and unpleasant conversations down through fear and intimidation, whereas in a 'nice' culture power is used covertly to stop people engaging in conflict because they want to belong to the 'in-group' and not make trouble.[64]

An important component of becoming and being a leader involves a redefining of your role as a follower. Being able to follow 'well' is vital as leaders need the support of those above them and they also need to influence their leaders when needed. This might involve 'upwards' delegation — *'taking the problem to the problem owner'* — knowing when your boss needs to deal with something instead of trying to deal with it yourself. A useful model to help leaders work out what needs to be done in various situations and who should do it is a responsibility assignment tool, a RACI matrix.[66] RACI stands for Responsible (who is responsible for doing the activity); Accountable (who has overall accountability); Consulted (who provides and who needs to be given information — a two-way process); Informed (who needs to be told what is going on — a one-way process).

Coping With and Managing Change

Part of being resilient and 'gritty' is coping with change. This involves both a psychological aspect and a more technical aspect. All change, even a positive change, involves some loss — both of competence (as you learn new skills or about a new environment) and of what you had before. It can be helpful to envision the changed, improved future, accept that any change takes time and that you might go through the stages of loss and grief (e.g. frustration, anger or withdrawal). Leaders therefore need to be able to recognise and acknowledge the psychological aspects of change in order to cope with their (what might be unexpected) feelings, as well as manage the transition process. Research into bereavement and grieving sheds an interesting light on this. For example, Klass et al.[67] suggests that instead of thinking of death as a complete ending, it might be helpful to maintain a continuing bond with the deceased person. It might be helpful therefore for Dr Gina to not see the move into a new role as a complete loss of what went before, but instead an opportunity to take forward and grow and develop existing relationships and experiences.

Being able to manage and lead change is one of the hallmarks of successful leaders, and leaders who can adapt well to changing circumstances tend to be more long-lasting. Alongside the psychological aspects of change, leaders need technical skills. A large number of change management tools and techniques are available, which can be helpful to use in curriculum design, development and delivery.[68] We can divide change initiatives and techniques into three types: linear (useful for technical change, project planning and management), iterative (changes which require some revisiting and which do not have a clear path) and complex change. Change leaders will need to use different approaches depending on the scale, time frame and complexity of the task. Project management tools are useful for physical or building projects (e.g. moving offices) and curriculum implementation (e.g. timetabling and allocating resources). For change projects at an earlier stage, which involve more people and complexity, models such as Kotter's '8 steps' help provide a checklist against which change projects can be planned and analysed.[69] These models emphasise the importance of engaging stakeholders at an early stage, setting and communicating a vision and empowering people to take action and deliver the change.

Kotter[69] also emphasises the importance of embedding the change in culture, so that people don't revert to the old ways. This involves a leader developing a deep understanding of the formal and informal organisations in which they work. The formal aspect includes the structure (who does what and who reports to whom), policies and procedures and the 'front face' of the organisation. The informal or hidden aspects include the culture (the 'way we do things round here') and sub-cultures (professional and departmental 'tribes and territories'); politics and power structures; values and beliefs; history and stories; and rituals, routines and symbols. '*Bolman and Deal*[70] *suggest that change leaders need to step back and take different perspectives or 'reframe', so as to help them see the organisation or change process from different people's points of view.... the four frames are structural, human resource, political and symbolic. Reframing can help explain why things are happening as they are, and help leaders devise new ways of working by 'looking through different lenses' to view what is happening*'[68] (p. 3). This would also reflect what Senge[71] calls a 'learning organisation', where leaders develop personal mastery, shared mental models and vision, team learning and systems thinking.

When developing and implementing change across organisations or systems, for example, a new health professions' curriculum, we cannot ignore the complexity. Such a programme operates across multiple organisations, involves many stakeholders, and needs to function on both the education and health systems. Complexity theories can help our understanding, suggesting that leaders need to use 'cognitive complexity' and systems thinking to think in multiple dimensions and relationships, use their networks, recognise ambiguity, and connect people, processes, tool and goals. An adaptive leader will be able to step back and see a system as complex ('get off the dance floor and onto the balcony' and back again), set boundaries, define simple rules and create the conditions for change[72] rather than attempting to 'manage' the change. Stacey suggests that working in the complex zone involves high uncertainty about the change and its implications and/or disagreement about what should be done. Whilst leaders can stimulate change by introducing uncertainty or disagreement into a process (perturbing the edge of chaos), in order to embed the change, they need to work with stakeholders to bring the change into the complicated or simple zones, so it can be managed.[73]

Summary

In this chapter, we have expanded some of the theories and models in relation to developing appropriate leadership skills and approaches. At the heart of this is understanding yourself, your strengths and weaknesses, and developing an open mindset that enables you to build fruitful relationships with others (your leaders and followers). Followers need to be able to trust and respect their leader, and part of this is meeting their expectations of what leaders do and say. So leaders need to demonstrate enough professional credibility and be aware of the power they have, drawn from a number of sources including the position they hold and their expertise. Being able to communicate well and openly with your teams and individuals is essential and, when good relationships are formed, then the leader is starting to build a culture, which can allow conflicts to occur and be safely resolved. Finally, we considered that leaders need to be comfortable with and be able to manage change, for themselves and for those around them.

Practice Highlights

- Leaders need to work on developing productive and meaningful relationships with their followers
- Followers need to be able to respect and trust their leaders, therefore leaders need to have credibility
- Understanding yourself is essential to becoming and being a good leader
- Leaders and followers both have a role in developing and maintaining a safe culture and climate

Chapter 3: How? — How To Use These Tools/Skills?

> ### Scenario
> Dr Gina has learned a lot now in terms of the skills and strengths she already has and has identified a number of gaps in her understanding and knowledge. She is feeling much more positive and is keen to start to apply her learning and new skills to different situations.

In this chapter, we take a number of situations, theories, models and 'learning lessons' and discuss how these can be applied in practice.

'Learning Leadership'

Starting at the top right petal of the 'Daffodil', leadership development can be carried out in undergraduate programmes, during postgraduate training and as part of continuing professional development (CPD). As we've said, leadership theories, practice and development can be broadly divided into three levels[34]: **intrapersonal** — this is about getting to know yourself, developing self-insight, understanding your strengths and weaknesses and your responses under pressure; **interpersonal** — this involves working in teams, with other people, patients, colleagues, learning how you are seen by others through conversation and feedback. At the **organisational or system level**, leadership involves learning about and understanding the wider systems and organisations in which you work, politics, processes and how change and quality/service improvement may be managed.

So, how do we 'learn leadership'? We think there are three ways: **formal opportunities**, such as short courses, workshops and longer, award-bearing programmes and through **practice**, obtaining constructive **feedback** and purposeful **reflection**. Learning leadership is a lifelong endeavour: good leaders have learned from their **experiences** and gained **practical wisdom** (phronesis) about how to behave and function in different situations. Petrie looks at this a slightly different way, suggesting we need **'horizontal leadership'**, which gives you an evidence base (in terms of theories, concepts, models and tools) about what leadership is, how it works and ways of approaching situations or tasks. However, as we said above, you can only really learn for yourself how to lead, follow and manage effectively, Petrie calls this **'vertical leadership'**, which comprises three elements: meeting challenges ('heat experiences'); 'sense-making' of the experience (through reflection and conversation) and being open to 'colliding perspectives' about what is going on.[74]

Reframing and Support

Talking with a colleague, Dr Gina commented that she now realised just how much of an educational leader's work is management. But management skills can be learned, and she was actually now looking forward to learning how to develop a 'Learning and Teaching Strategic Plan', using project management techniques to map out, prioritise and delegate activities, drawing on her previous course review experience. Dr Gina also reflected that she has started to feel more confident that she could do the job, but that she needed to continue to build her confidence: 'do some small things well'. From a leadership perspective, she feels like a servant leader, not in the role for 'quick wins' but to make a difference and leave a legacy. She also realised that her 'grit' and resilience contributed to this feeling, she is passionate about education but had got ground down in everyday pressures; once she had got those under control, she could think more strategically and focus on the 'long game'.

Dr Gina started to realise that she already had a lot of 'leadership skills' but had never really thought of herself as a senior leader. One of her colleagues on the leadership course had suggested that Dr Gina should find a mentor, a 'wise counsel'. Everyone needs support in a new role, and a 'guide on the side', whether a trusted peer, coach or mentor, can really help provide an outside perspective and ideas about different issues.[75] A work 'buddy' can act as a critical friend to give you support and feedback on how you are performing. Through finding a mentor and working with her course group, she began to reframe her ideas of what leadership and leaders mean. Before Dr Gina had thought and learned about leadership, she had held a very traditional view — thinking of leaders as big 'L' leaders who were often 'great men', or had very senior positions.[76] She had also thought of 'management' as something that was a bit on the 'dark side', and certainly inferior to leadership. And she had never heard about followership. This mindset shift was instrumental in helping her to understand that an individual's credibility, personal power and influence results from a host of factors. Simply being in a senior position does not make you a good leader and conversely, you can be a very effective 'little "l"' leader.[39]

Dr Gina was invited to join an informal group comprising the other Deans of Learning and Teaching in the University. At first she was reluctant, feeling that she would just be revealing her lack of knowledge, but her mentor encouraged her, explaining the importance of networking and collaboration to educational leaders. She was surprised to find not only that the group was very welcoming but also that they were very impressed that she was a senior clinician and had carried out a major curriculum review. She realised that she was not alone in feeling like an 'imposter' and that most of the other Deans had also felt very out of their depth when they started in role.[77,78] This was why they had formed this informal group where they could share ideas, but also get support and ask one another what they felt might be stupid questions. One of the other experienced Deans offered to let Dr Gina 'shadow' her so that she could learn more about the universities' policies and procedures, another suggested that she offer to join one of the University's working parties on curriculum development or review. She also learned about another informal group, which was specifically for women in the University, a 'Lean-In group', to share issues and strategies relating to gender issues. She had never realised that all these development opportunities existed, it was collaborative, shared and distributed leadership in action.

Letting Go

Following a useful conversation with one of the other Deans, who was astounded that Dr Gina managed to work clinically in addition to the Dean role, Dr Gina decided to talk with her manager, the Head of School, about her workload. She had realised that it was not that her time management was poor, it was just that the workload was too much, and 'you can't do everything'. Rather than continue to struggle on, she had come to appreciate that she needed to give some things up.[79] A key issue for clinicians is that because their personal and social identity is closely tied up with their professional identity of 'being', for example, a doctor, nurse or physiotherapist, it is a huge identity shift to even contemplate giving up clinical work, as this is such a central part of identity. Making this decision is therefore difficult, and so because Dr Gina was aware of this, she had decided to cut down her clinical work first, rather than stopping entirely and moving into the School full-time.

Before her meeting with the Head of School, she worked with her mentor to clarify what she wanted to get out of the meeting; what her main interests were; where she saw her contribution to the School, in the short and medium term; and the formal professional development she needed to equip her for the new role. This structured and proactive approach resulted in a very productive meeting in which they set SMART (Specific, Measurable, Achievable, Realistic, Timebound) objectives for Dr Gina for the next 18 months. As part of this, they agreed that Dr Gina would drop one day clinically for the next year and then this would be reviewed; that she would undertake a one-day project management course and a one-day strategic planning course, and be nominated for the University Senior Leaders' programme; and that a part-time administrator would be allocated to her, to help with the day-to-day administration and paperwork. The Head of School reinforced to Gina that he felt she had done a great job on the curriculum review, he appreciated that there were other priorities at the moment, but that once these had been addressed, she could take on another similar project as he had every confidence in her. He also said to her to ask him or the other senior team if she needed help, that their door was always open. She came out of the meeting feeling much more valued, positive, empowered and supported, and much more appreciative of her Head of School's leadership and management skills and abilities.

Developing the Team

Learning about leadership and followership, and the different leadership approaches and styles was really helpful for Dr Gina. Developing her own self-insight and understanding her drivers, strengths and weaknesses is essential (as is management and planning of activities), but she cannot lead all these activities without the input and support of individuals and teams. One of the most powerful things Dr Gina learned was the importance of being 'yourself' — authentic leadership. Of course you have to know yourself to be your 'best' self, but what followers want from their leader is to feel valued, included, stretched and supported. From an inclusive leadership perspective, 'making a difference' as a leader involves including and empowering others to make that difference, not necessarily doing everything yourself. Healthcare and educational work involves service (servant leadership); values and morals (value-led and moral leadership); people (person-led leadership); caring (caring and compassionate leadership) and collaboration (collaborative, distributed and shared leadership). And whilst a leader sometimes needs to take a different style in certain situations (such as authoritative or directive), it is these underpinning approaches that need to be aligned with the work being done, the people involved, the ethos and culture of organisations and the values and beliefs of the leader themselves. Articulating and living the values setting the culture are all examples of authentic leadership in action.

Dr Gina decided that she would put her learning into practice and introduce her two main teams to some self- and team development activities. Her aim was to build the culture of psychological safety and help team members understand one another better in terms of their strengths and weaknesses, so the members could help one another compensate for these; to have some fun so team members would bond better and become more resilient, and to develop a common 'language' to describe people's preferences and different ways of working. She decided to use different approaches with each team. The School Learning and Teaching team was a new team that Dr Gina had established to support her in her new role and many of the members were unfamiliar to Dr Gina. She decided to start with asking members to undertake a Belbin Team Role Inventory.[59] This was really helpful both to Dr Gina and to the team, as they realised they had a good spread of team role preferences across the 'thinking', 'action' and 'social' domains, and the members really enjoyed learning about themselves and others. As a result, the team worked together to plan their activities for the next year, with people offering to take on various elements based on their role preferences. The Programme

Directors' team was well-established and Dr Gina knew most of them from her previous role fairly well. She asked a trained MBTI facilitator to carry out a Myers Briggs Type Indicator (MBTI™) test with each of them and then work with them as a group to learn more about the way they saw the world, and the way they liked to work. They already had clear roles and she felt that a Belbin Team Role Inventory would not give as much useful information. Following this, she could see that the team members appeared more appreciative of one another, had a common language to use and were reflecting on their decision-making differently. Both teams wanted to undertake more development as a team, and valued that Dr Gina had given them the opportunity for this professional development.

The Wider Picture

Dr Gina realised, whilst attending some of the senior meetings for the first time that, although she already knew a lot about her 'industry', there were some gaps in her knowledge and understanding. Taking on board the helpful 'positive self-talk' mantra, '*you can't know what you don't know*', she decided to learn more about how funding and quality systems worked across education and healthcare by asking her Head of School who she could talk to, and where she could find out the information she needed. He offered to introduce her to the Director of Education in the main teaching hospital so she could learn about the healthcare setting and ask the Head of Quality at the University if they would send Dr Gina some useful documents and if she could spend some time observing their work, committees and processes.

Dr Gina had learned about a number of change management techniques on the course, and whilst she had really enjoyed leading on the review of the nursing curriculum, had done this without any formal training or development. She had already established two teams, which would help her plan and take programme changes forward and she decided to work with them to develop the Learning and Teaching Strategic Plan, starting with developing and setting out a shared vision. She felt this would help establish an inclusive culture and demonstrate to her teams that she valued their ideas, perspectives and input, and would help share the power amongst the teams, rather than her taking an authoritative approach and using her positional power. She knew that the accountability lay with her, but (drawing on the RACI model) that the responsibility needed to be shared between the team members. She also wanted to use her 'cognitive complexity' in that, whilst she was starting to see the whole picture from a systems perspective herself ('from the balcony'), she knew that she needed the teams to come to some agreement and certainty, so that the vision could be translated into a Strategic and Operational plan, which could be implemented from the complicated and simple zones. She wanted the teams to have a 'quick visible win'[69] to keep them motivated as there were no real external pressures upon them, so she asked them to identify some short courses or activities that could be carried out this year.

Paying it Forward: Embedding Leadership into Curricula and Professional Development

As you can see, our understanding of leadership is constantly shifting: it is not a static concept. Over the last few years, many health professionals and educators have become more politicised and we see a current shift in the way doctors and health professionals see themselves as leaders, combining **accountability, advocacy** and **activism**. This involves putting core values into action and incorporating these into everyday behaviours. Table 4 sets out the three areas (Column 1) and describes how these might be displayed in action (Column 2). Training and education will need to be provided in various topics to encourage these values (listed in Column 3), and from a leadership perspective, we have highlighted some of the leadership theories or approaches that underpin these activities (Column 4). These three areas do not necessarily relate to undergraduate, postgraduate and continuing professional development, or to levels of seniority, but there is a developmental aspect to this, and it starts with accountability.

Summary

Dr Gina has now been Dean of Learning and Teaching for 5 years. In that time she has learned a lot about herself and the organisation is working well with an expanded team across the School on many new projects, and is mentoring some of the less experienced staff, developing them as 'little "l" leaders'. With a lot of sadness she gave up her clinical work 3 years ago, but it meant she could focus on the development of new programmes for the School including a distance-learning masters' degree and a Physician Associate programme. She has developed a *'health professions' leadership and management'* curriculum, which is now embedded into all the programmes and has received national acclaim. She was recently approached by two junior members of staff to mentor them, so they could be prepared to be able to move into leadership positions for the future. Occasionally she still feels a bit like an 'imposter', and certainly not the expert people seem to think she is, but most of the time she loves her work and feels she is working at the right level. She is so pleased she didn't give up all those years ago, and is very grateful to all her colleagues who supported and mentored her into becoming a health professions' education leader.

Table 4.   Leadership development activities.

	Core values in action	Education/training in …	Leadership theory/approaches
Accountability *These values in action and training should be part of every undergraduate and postgraduate curriculum*	➤ For care of individual patients ➤ Requires clinical expertise, care and compassion ➤ For own professional conduct/clinical practice ➤ For patient safety at individual level ➤ Responsibility for self-care	➤ Clinical knowledge and expertise ➤ Communication skills ➤ Professionalism, role boundaries ➤ Self-development, self-insight ➤ Time and stress management ➤ Teamwork ➤ Patient safety	➤ Caring & compassionate leadership ➤ Resilience/grit/EI/ ➤ Emotional well-being ➤ Followership
Advocacy *To advocate effectively for students, colleagues, patients, healthcare and education, you need a deeper understanding of the context and cultures, plus skills to navigate, persuade and influence for change*	➤ Patient advocacy ➤ Health advocacy ➤ Community advocacy ➤ Challenging decisions ➤ Quality/service improvements ➤ Social accountability ➤ Interprofessional/ ➤ Multidisciplinary team working ➤ Preventive care, public health perspective ➤ Care of others (patients, colleagues and learners)	➤ Service and organisational systems, structures, functions and funding ➤ Public health and preventive care ➤ Integrated service approaches ➤ Conflict resolution ➤ Negotiation, persuasion and influencing skills ➤ Leadership and followership	➤ Dispersed/distributed leadership ➤ Shared/collaborative leadership ➤ Inclusive leadership ➤ Relational leadership ➤ Compassionate/caring leadership

Activism *Not everyone will (or should?) become an activist, but when we feel very strongly, sometimes we have to put our heads above the parapet and work actively with power and politics in complex systems*	➤ Increased politicisation
	➤ Willingness to become involved
	➤ Challenging 'authority'
	➤ Whistle-blowing
		➤ Diversity, inclusivity and unconscious bias
		➤ Power dynamics
		➤ Political awareness and astuteness
		➤ Strategic management
		➤ Systems thinking and complexity science
		➤ Value-based healthcare
			➤ Inclusive leadership
			➤ Collective leadership
			➤ Complexity and systems thinking
			➤ Adaptive leadership
			➤ Servant leadership:
			  ☐ legacy building
			  ☐ Stewardship

Practice Highlights

- Leadership learning is a lifelong endeavour: development happens through a combination of formal learning, experience and reflection
- Having support from colleagues and building a network helps provide perspective on what leadership actually involves
- Moving into a new position or role usually involves giving something up — this can be difficult
- Building a strong team, which values diverse ideas and perspectives is also vital
- Leadership and management are starting to be embedded into health professions' curricula at all levels

References

1. Storey J. *Leadership in Organizations: Current Issues and Key Trends*. 3rd ed. London: Routledge; 2016.

2. Kok J, Van den Heuvel S. Leading in a VUCA World. Springer; 2018.

3. Frank JR, Snell L, Sherbino J. *CanMEDS 2015 Physician Competency Framework*. Ottawa: Royal College of Physicians and Surgeons of Canada; 2015.

4. McKimm J, O'Sullivan H. When I say… leadership. *Medical Education*. 2016;50(9):896–7.

5. Drucker P. *Management Challenges for the 21st Century*. New York: Libro Editorial Harper Business; 1999.

6. Mowbray D. Leader workstyle that stimulates positive psychological health and safety at work Management Advisory Service; 2019.

7. Denhardt JV, Denhardt RB. *The New Public Service: Serving, Not Steering*. Armonk, NY: ME Sharpe; 2003.

8. Lewin K. The research center for group dynamics at Massachusetts Institute of Technology. *Sociometry*. 1945;8(2):126–36.

9. Fiedler FE. Validation and extension of the contingency model of leadership effectiveness: A review of empirical findings. *Psychological Bulletin*. 1971;76(2):128.

10. Hersey P, Blanchard KH, Natemeyer WE. Situational leadership, perception, and the impact of power. *Group & Organization Studies*. 1979;4(4):418–28.

11. Kouzes JM, Posner BZ. *The Student Leadership Challenge: Five Practices for Becoming an Exemplary Leader*. John Wiley & Sons; 2018.

12. Nonaka I, Takeuchi H. The wise leader. *Harvard Business Review*. 2011;89(5):58–67.

13. Schippers M. Ikigai: Reflection on life goals optimizes performance and happiness; 2017.

14. Mohammed M, Thomas K. Enabling community and trust: Shared leadership for collective creativity. *The Foundation Review*. 2014;6(4):10.

15. Sinek S. The golden circle. Gumroad com; 2015. Accessed from: http://tinyurl.com/golden-circle-sinek

16. Duckworth, A. *Grit: The Power of Passion and Perseverance*. New York: Scribner; 2016.

17. Barrow M, McKimm J, Gasquoine S. The policy and the practice: Early-career doctors and nurses as leaders and followers in the delivery of health care. *Advances in Health Sciences Education*. 2011;16(1):17–29.

18. Souba, WW. The being of leadership. *Philosophy, Ethics, and Humanities in Medicine*. 2011;6(1):5.

19. McKenna B, Rooney D. Wise leadership and the capacity for ontological acuity. *Management Communication Quarterly*. 2008;21(4):537–46.

20. Greenleaf RK. *Servant Leadership: A Journey into the Nature of Legitimate Power and Greatness*. Paulist Press; 2002.

21. Bass BM, Bass Bernard M. *Leadership and Performance Beyond Expectations*. New York: The Free Press; 1985.

22. Cardiff S, McCormack B, McCance T. Person-centred leadership: A relational approach to leadership derived through action research. *Journal of Clinical Nursing*. 2018;27(15–16):3056–69.

23. Hollander EP. *Inclusive Leadership*. Taylor & Francis; 2009.

24. Gabriel Y. The caring leader — What followers expect of their leaders and why? *Leadership*. 2015;11(3):316–34.

25. West MA, Chowla R. *Compassionate Leadership for Compassionate Health Care*. Compassion: Routledge; 2017:237–57.

26. de Zulueta PC. Developing compassionate leadership in health care: An integrative review. *Journal of Healthcare Leadership*. 2016;8:1.

27. Western S. *Leadership: A Critical Text*. SAGE Publications Limited; 2019.

28. Nations U. Sustainable Development Goals United States of America; 2015. Available from: https://www.un.org/sustainabledevelopment/sustainable-development-goals/.

29. Griggs D, Stafford-Smith M, Gaffney O, Rockstrom J, Ohman MC, Shyamsundar P, et al. Policy: Sustainable development goals for people and planet. *Nature*. 2013;495(7441):305–7.

30. Lichtenstein BB, Uhl-Bien, Marion R, Seers A, Orton JD, & Schreiber C. Complexity leadership theory: An interactive perspective on leading in complex adaptive systems. *Management Department Faculty Publications*. 2006;8(4):2–12.

31. Obolensky N. *Complex Adaptive Leadership: Embracing Paradox and Uncertainty*. Routledge; 2017.

32. Heifetz RA, Heifetz R, Grashow A, Linsky M. *The Practice of Adaptive Leadership: Tools and Tactics for Changing Your Organization and the World*. Boston: Harvard Business Press; 2009.

33. Bolman LG, Gallos JV. *Reframing Academic Leadership*. San Francisco: John Wiley & Sons; 2010.

34. McKimm J, Swanwick T. Faculty development for leadership development. In Steinert Y, editor. *Faculty Development in the Health Professions: A Focus on Research and Practice*. Springer Netherlands; 2014:XVII, 442.

35. Gorsky D, Mann K, Sargeant J. *Project Management and Leadership: Practical Tips for Medical School Leaders.* MedEdPublish; 2016;5(3):41.

36. Gosling J, Mintzberg H. The five minds of a manager. *Harvard Business Review.* 2003;81(11):54–63.

37. Lieff S, Albert M. What do we do? Practices and learning strategies of medical education leaders. *Medical Teacher.* 2012;34(4):312–9.

38. Uhl-Bien M, Riggio RE, Lowe KB, Carsten MK. Followership theory: A review and research agenda. *The Leadership Quarterly.* 2014;25(1):83–104.

39. Kelley RE. Rethinking followership. In: Riggio RE, Chaleff I, Lipman-Blume J, editors. *The Art of Followership: How Great Followers Create Great Leaders and Organizations.* Jossey-Bass; 2008:5–16.

40. Kellerman B. *Followership: How Followers are Creating Change and Changing Leaders.* Boston: Harvard Business School Press; 2008.

41. Riggio RE, Chaleff I, Lipman-Blumen J. *The Art of Followership: How Great Followers Create Great Leaders and Organizations.* San Francisco: John Wiley & Sons; 2008; 146.

42. DeRue DS, Ashford SJ. Who will lead and who will follow? A social process of leadership identity construction in organizations. *Academy of Management Review.* 2010;35(4):627–47.

43. Tee EY, Paulsen N, Ashkanasy NM. Revisiting followership through a social identity perspective: The role of collective follower emotion and action. *The Leadership Quarterly.* 2013;24(6):902–18.

44. Epitropaki O, Kark R, Mainemelis C, Lord RG. Leadership and followership identity processes: A multilevel review. *The Leadership Quarterly.* 2017;28(1):104–29.

45. Paulhus DL, Williams KM. The dark triad of personality: Narcissism, Machiavellianism, and psychopathy. *Journal of Research in Personality.* 2002;36(6):556–63.

46. Seligman M, Flourish P. A visionary new understanding of happiness and well-being. *Policy.* 2011;27(3):60–1.

47. Dweck CS, Yeager DS. The psychology of thinking about the future. In: Oettingen G, Sevincer AT, Gollwitzer, editor. *Mindsets Change the Imagined and Actual Future.* New York: Guilfor Press; 2018:362.

48. Bohmer R. Leadership with a small "l". *BMJ.* 2010;340:c483.

49. Mills J, McKimm J. Resilience: Why it matters and how doctors can improve it. *British Journal of Hospital Medicine.* 2016;77(11):630–3.

50. Mintz LJ, Stoller JK. A systematic review of physician leadership and emotional intelligence. *Journal of Graduate Medical Education.* 2014;6(1):21–31.

51. Goleman DBR, Davidson RJ, Druskat V, Kohlrieser G. *Building Blocks of Emotional Intelligence.* Florence, MA: More Than Sound, LLC; 2017.

52. Salovey P, Mayer JD. Emotional intelligence. *Imagination, Cognition and Personality.* 1990;9(3):185–211.

53. Petrides KV, Mikolajczak M, Mavroveli S, Sanchez-Ruiz MJ, Furnham A, Pérez-González JC. Developments in trait emotional intelligence research. *Emotion Review.* 2016;8(4):335–41.

54. Rock D. The neuroscience of leadership (Doctoral dissertation, Middlesex University). 2010.

55. McKimm J, Forrest K, Thistlethwaite J. *Medical Education at a Glance*. Hoboken: John Wiley & Sons; 2017.

56. Kaufman SB, Yaden DB, Hyde E, Tsukayama E. The light vs. dark triad of personality: Contrasting two very different profiles of human nature. *Frontiers in Psychology*. 2019;10:467.

57. Kouzes JM, Posner BZ. Leadership begins with an inner journey. *Leader to Leader*. 2011;2011(60):22–7.

58. Tuckman BW. *Educational Psychology: From Theory to Application*. Harcourt Brace Jovanovich; 1992.

59. Belbin RM. *Team Roles at Work*. Routledge; 2012.

60. Coyle D. *The Culture Code: The Secrets of Highly Successful Groups*. Bantam; 2018.

61. Brown B. *Daring Greatly: How the Courage to be Vulnerable Transforms the Way We Live, Love, Parent, and Lead*. Penguin; 2015.

62. Brown B. *Brené Brown: The Power of Vulnerability*. TED; 2010.

63. Brown B. *Dare to Lead: Brave Work. Tough Conversations. Whole Hearts*. Random House; 2018.

64. Perks-Baker Susie FB. From nasty to nice and back again: Seven tips for encouraging cognitive diversity; 2019. Available from: https://www.kingsfund.org.uk/blog/2019/01/encouraging-cognitive-diversity.

65. Raven BH. A power/interaction model of interpersonal influence: French and Raven thirty years later. *Journal of Social Behavior & Personality*. 1992;7;217.

66. Hambleton L. *Treasure Chest of Six Sigma Growth Methods, Tools, and Best Practices: A Desk Reference Book for Innovation and Growth*. Upper Saddle River, NJ: Prentice Hall; 2008.

67. Klass D, Silverman PR, Nickman S. *Continuing Bonds: New Understandings of Grief*. Washington, DC: Taylor & Francis; 1996.

68. McKimm J, Jones PK. Twelve tips for applying change models to curriculum design, development and delivery. *Medical Teacher*. 2018;40(5):520–6.

69. Kotter J. *The 8-Step Process for Leading Change*. Kotter International; 2012.

70. Lee G. Bolman TED. *Reframing Organizations: Artistry, Choice, and Leadership*. New Jersey: Jossey-Bass, A John Wiley & Sons, Inc.; 2017:512.

71. Senge PM. *The Fifth Discipline Fieldbook: Strategies and Tools for Building a Learning Organization*. Crown Business; 2014.

72. Heifetz R, Grashow A, Linsky M. Leadership in a (permanent) crisis. *Harvard Business Review*. 2009;87(7–8):62–9, 153.

73. Stacey RD. *Complex Responsive Processes in Organisations: Learning and Knowledge Creation*. London: Routledge; 2001.

74. Petrie, N. *Vertical Leadership Development — Part 1: Developing Leader for a Complex World*. Center for Creative Leadership; 2014. Accessed from: http://insights. ccl. org/wp-content/uploads/2015/04/VerticalLeadersPart1. pdf.

75. McKimm J, O'Sullivan H. Leadership, management and mentoring: Applying theory to practice. In: Cleland J, Durning SJ, editors. *Researching Medical Education*, chap. 23. John Wiley & Sons; 2015:269.

76. Slootweg IA, van der Vleuten C, Heineman MJ, Scherpbier A, Lombarts KM. Program directors in their role as leaders of teaching teams in residency training. *Medical Teacher*. 2014;36(12):1073–9.

77. McKimm J. *Developing Tomorrow's Leaders in Health and Social Care Education: Case Studies in Leadership in Medical and Health Care Education*. Higher Education Academy; 2004.

78. Bassaw B. Determinants of successful deanship. *Medical Teacher*. 2010;32(12):1002–6.

79. Lieff S, Banack JGP, Baker L, Martimianakis MA, Verma S, Whiteside C, et al. Understanding the needs of department chairs in academic medicine. *Academic Medicine*. 2013;88(7):960–6.

FUTURE DIRECTIONS — WHERE ARE WE HEADING?

Gary D. Rogers and W. David Carr

Scenario

Year: 2030. Venue: Health School of the Future. Time: 0730 hours.

Third-year health student Yu Yan is woken by gentle music newly composed to meet her tastes by her Personalised Augmented Tutor (PAT), who also reminds her of her learning plan for the day. Over breakfast she asks PAT to display her recent clinical informatics notes, which she reviews in preparation for an assessment later in the week.

When she arrives at school, she enters the simulation centre, dons a sleek pair of augmented reality (AR) glasses and joins a small group of colleagues from multiple health professions with whom she has been learning for several weeks as part of an interprofessional education team. As they move around the centre in a simulated ward round, the members of the team interact with a mixture of AR avatars and live simulated patients (SPs). The avatars exhibit realistic physical signs and provide responses to their straight-forward questions driven by artificial intelligence (AI) systems and the SPs provide more nuanced responses that test the quality of the students' human capabilities.

At the end of the session, Yu Yan participates in a summative assessment where she is required to obtain a history from and examine an AR avatar, consult imaging guidelines, order appropriate investigations, then interpret the results provided by AI reports. She checks the latest online treatment recommendations and seeks advice on how to find the answer to a particular management question from her clinical informatics instructor via video link. She records her recommendations in a simulated electronic health record, which connects to further AI systems that determine their appropriateness to the situation, thus assessing her cognitive domain learning. She then explains the diagnosis and recommended treatment to a live SP, with the same face and clothing as the avatar, who assesses the effectiveness of her interpersonal communication. Subsequently, as part of the recommended management, she undertakes a clinical procedure using a physical part-task trainer, which is overlaid in her glasses with an AR image of the whole patient to enhance the authenticity of her learning experience. The trainer is equipped with electronic motion and pressure sensors whose signals are combined with the video feed from her AR glasses to enable another AI algorithm to assess the quality of her developing psychomotor skills.

Later in the day, she reflects on her experiences in the simulation with her interprofessional colleagues and a facilitator then completes a video journal, which the facilitator subsequently assesses for evidence of learning in the affective domain using a validated methodology.

Introduction

There is no doubt that practice in the health professions will change dramatically in the next decade and the rate of such change appears to be accelerating. Historically, health professional education has been slow to respond to changes in practice and developments in educational methodology. However, as educators, we have both an opportunity and a responsibility to anticipate changes to the ways that healthcare, social care and health promotion will be enacted and to modify our educational practices in order to ensure that they will continue to be fit for purpose.

In this section, we will consider some of the most likely directions in which health practice will change in the next decade and beyond, the modified educational approaches that will be required in order to equip graduates for these changes and new learning methodologies that will allow these modified approaches to be implemented. In Chapter 1, each particular area of anticipated practice change will be considered under a numbered heading. We will also look at the educational implications of these changes, across the health professions and across the three domains of learning in Bloom's time-honoured taxonomy: cognitive, psychomotor and affective.[1] In Chapters 2 and 3, we will discuss the new or modified educational approaches that will need to be developed in response to each area of anticipated practice change (Chapter 2), as well as exploring emerging and anticipated learning methodologies that might enable us to implement these adjustments effectively (Chapter 3). Across the three chapters, we will utilise a common numbering system to identify the thread of discussion following from each anticipated health practice change identified in this chapter, as summarized in Table 1.

Table 1. Development of threads of discussion consequent upon each anticipated change in health professional practice.

	Chapter 1: Why? (Anticipated changes in health professional practice)	Chapter 2: What? (New educational approaches required)	Chapter 3: How? (New learning methodologies to allow implementation)
1	Increasing complexity and recognition of the determinants of health	Interprofessional education	'Second generation' interprofessional education
2	Practitioner distress	Building personal resilience	New ways to build human capabilities and personal resilience in practitioners
3	Developments in artificial intelligence and robotics	New and reprioritised professional capabilities	Innovations to enable acquisition of new and reprioritised capabilities
4	Ready access to 'just-in-time' factual information	Authentic assessment of learning outcomes	Enhanced assessment methodologies
5	Increased reliance on complex technology	Information technology literacy	Gaining information technology literacy

Chapter 1: Why?

This chapter will describe some of the most important changes in health professional practice that appear likely to occur over the next decade and beyond, as well as the implications of these anticipated changes for health professional education.

1. Increasing Complexity and Recognition of the Determinants of Health

Population profiles are aging rapidly in developed countries and are also projected to do so in developing countries in the coming years.[2] These demographic changes are associated with a shift in the most prominent health problems facing societies from acute presentations of single diseases or injuries towards multiple morbidity, chronicity and complexity of treatment and prevention requirements.[3,4] These changes are impacting significantly on how health funds are spent[5] and on the working life of health practitioners.[6] They necessitate increased attention to the importance of health practitioners acquiring highly developed human capabilities, in addition to scientific understanding and technical skills, if they are to be effective in their work.[7]

Further, since the landmark findings of the Black Report[8] and the Whitehall Study[9] in the United Kingdom, we have increasingly come to understand how health outcomes in human populations are shaped by socio-economic position. More recent work by Krieger[10] and many others have shown how other social determinants such as sexism, racial discrimination, homophobia, working conditions, globalisation and urbanisation form a complex web of causation of the world's most significant health problems.[11] The serious expected health impacts of environmental degradation, particularly climate change, are also likely to be amplified in the decades ahead.[12] The importance of addressing the interplay of social and environmental determinants in both the primary and secondary prevention of illness will add further complexity to the daily practice of health and social care professionals.

In all healthcare settings, but especially in acute hospitals, the 'wicked' problem of patient safety remains only partially addressed[13] and the increasing prevalence of multiple morbidity and complexity of care seem likely to make this issue still harder to tackle into the future. Inquiries into prominent instances of healthcare misadventure in multiple countries over an extended period have pointed to problems with communication and collaboration between health professionals as significant causative factors.[14-16]

As healthcare and health promotion become more complex into the future, for the reasons outlined, the skills and knowledges of a range of practitioners from different health and social care professions will increasingly be required to optimise outcomes for individuals and communities. These professionals will also need specific capacities to enable them to collaborate and coordinate their practice to enhance its effectiveness and the safety of their patients and clients. These *interprofessional* collaborative practice capabilities are additional to profession-specific competencies, much as musicians who seek to perform effectively in an orchestra need specific training and practice to do so, in addition to virtuosity on their own instrument.[17]

Interprofessional capabilities span all of the three domains of learning first suggested by Bloom et al.[1] In the cognitive domain, they include an understanding of the origins, philosophies and scopes of practice of each of the health professions with whom learners are likely to collaborate in future practice, as well as their own intended profession. This learning has been referred to as 'health professions literacy'.[18] Also in the cognitive domain, practitioners require an intellectual understanding of how teams work and how their effectiveness may be optimised.

Successful collaborative practice also requires a range of trainable skills that might be thought to reside in the *psychomotor* domain of Bloom's taxonomy. These include proficiency in communication (both between professionals and with patients, clients and their significant others), the synthesis of ideas from different perspectives and then negotiation of management plans between practitioners and with the people for whom they are caring. Trainable techniques for stress management, the de-escalation of heightened emotional states and the resolution of conflict might also be thought of as residing in this domain.

In the *affective* domain, interprofessional collaborative capabilities comprise acquisition of the values that the community expects of its health professionals under the so-called 'social contract'.[19] These include respect for persons (including students and practitioners in one's own and other professions, as well as for patients, clients and communities), personal responsibility and placing the welfare of others ahead of the practitioner's own interest.

Multiple frameworks of interprofessional collaborative practice capabilities have been developed around the world, but there is broad consensus about the key requirements and these have recently been synthesised into a common set of competencies by O'Keefe et al.[20]

2. Practitioner Distress

In the last few years, there has been increasing concern about distress and even suicide among health professionals, particularly those in their first few years of practice.[21-25] Many commentators have emphasised the likely relationship between these outcomes and avoidable factors such as supervisor bullying and excessive workloads.[24,26-28] There is no question that healthcare facilities of the future will need to eliminate these unconscionable workplace practices. Even when these reforms have been fully achieved, however, practice in the health professions will remain *inherently* stressful, dealing — as it often does — with life and death and encountering patients, clients and their significant others at some of the most difficult times of their lives.

Similarly, effective post-registration training and development of health professionals in their first few years of practice requires close supervision by more senior colleagues with the provision and receipt of clear feedback about their developing competence. Preparedness to seek feedback actively and respond to it positively is vitally important for health professionals in the early years after registration and indeed throughout their careers.[29] It is important that senior colleagues deliver feedback professionally and constructively, but, even in ideal circumstances, being informed that one's performance is not yet optimal remains confronting and requires a capacity to regulate one's emotional responses appropriately. Additionally, effective health practice often requires an ability to begin to work effectively when there is only an incomplete picture of the causes of the patient's or client's presenting problem. Sometimes a complete diagnostic explanation for the symptoms that the patient or client is experiencing cannot be found and yet health practitioners still need to be able to work with them constructively and provide helpful care.[30] Sitting comfortably with this uncertainty is particularly difficult for students during training and for newly graduated practitioners, providing another source of significant emotional stress.

The ability to respond positively and constructively to unavoidably stressful practice experiences is important for the interests of health professionals, but it is also critical to the welfare of their patients and clients. It is well-recognised that distressed practitioners are less empathetic and their clinical performance may suffer, potentially compromising patient and client safety.[23,24,31-34] This underlines the importance of developing educational approaches that assist health professional students to develop their ability to manage stress adaptively — their personal resilience[35] — in addition to strategies aimed at reducing avoidable workplace stresses, in order to protect the safety of both health professionals and the patients and clients they serve.

The increasing complexity and chronicity of the health problems facing humans, described under Part 1 of this chapter, appear likely to magnify the stress experienced by health professionals into the future. In this light, educational approaches aimed at building the personal resilience of health professional learners, which will be discussed in Chapters 2 and 3, can be expected to become even more important.

3. Developments in Artificial Intelligence and Robotics

The term 'artificial intelligence' (AI) was coined more than 60 years ago by US computer scientist John McCarthy,[36] based on earlier work by others including British mathematician Alan Turing and philosophical imagining that goes back at least as far as Descartes in the 17th century.[37] Many definitions have been proposed but, recently, Kaplan and Haenlein[38] have neatly characterised the phenomenon as 'a system's ability to correctly interpret external data, to learn from such data, and to use those learnings to achieve specific goals and tasks through flexible adaptation' (p. 15). The overarching term is often taken to include the concepts of 'machine learning', which is the ability of computers to learn from experience without being explicitly programmed;[39] and 'robotics', which is 'the branch of technology that deals with the design, construction, operation, and application of robots'.[40]

The first application of AI to healthcare may have been the 'MYCIN' system, developed in the mid-1970s to assist with selection of the most appropriate antibiotic regimen for a particular clinical situation, based on organism susceptibility, synergistic combinations, patient allergies and responses to prior therapy.[41] Since that time, and particularly in the last decade, the development of AI systems, based on machine learning, has expanded exponentially. Recently, they have been shown to be highly effective at diagnosing diabetic retinopathy from fundal photographs,[42] tuberculosis from plain chest X-rays[43] and to outperform most expert dermatologists in determining whether a photographed skin lesion is malignant or benign.[44]

The word 'robotics' was first coined by science fiction writer Isaac Asimov in 1941. Asimov also provided an early imagining of science's application to healthcare in the memorable short story *Segregationist*, set in a future where robots and humans are both treated as citizens.[45] Curiously, robots have taken to replacing parts of their bodies with synthetic organs derived from proteinaceous tissue, whereas humans have done the opposite, preferring to substitute dysfunctioning body parts with metal replacements. The story is told from the point of view of a surgeon who seeks, unsuccessfully, to persuade his patient — a senator — that replacement of the patient's heart with an organic alternative will provide the best outcomes. Despite the evidence, the patient chooses a mechanical heart because he believes it will be 'stronger'. The surgeon is accused by a colleague of being a 'segregationist' because he feels uncomfortable about the tendency of the two sentient life forms on the planet to merge with each other in this fashion. In a powerful closing scene, the surgeon places his hands into a hot oven to sterilise them prior to the procedure and is revealed to be a robot himself.

Surgery is the healthcare practice that has most utilised robot-like devices to date. The first 'robot-assisted' operation is generally considered to have been performed in 1985 by a neurosurgical team supported by Kwoh's group of biomedical engineers in Long Beach, California.[46] They utilised a robotic device to manipulate the instruments for stereotactic brain surgery very accurately, guided by computed tomography (CT) scanning. A wide range of surgical procedures has employed robotic instruments since.[47] In almost all of these cases, however, the instruments have been under the direct control of a human surgeon (albeit with augmented precision and, sometimes, from a remote location) rather than driven by the judgement of a computerised system, as envisaged by Asimov. Into the future, it can be expected that the fields of AI and robotics will converge in the surgical sphere, with robotic devices directed by computer systems to undertake procedures that they have themselves designed on the basis of a patient's pathological diagnosis.

Another potential area for development in robotic surgery is in the miniaturisation of autonomous robotic devices to the 'micro' or 'nano' scales so that they can be introduced into the body and travel to the site of disease through the circulatory system without damaging healthy tissue. Soto and Chrostowski[48] have suggested a wide range of healthcare applications for such devices.

The recent advent of practical AI-driven robots of humanoid form has led to investigation of the potential for their application to wider fields of health and social care. A recent report prepared by the UK Parliamentary Office of Science and Technology[49] suggests applications of these innovations in a broad range of areas, such as providing physical assistance and rehabilitation services to people who are frail, aged or with disabilities, social support to people who are isolated and cognitive assistance to people living with dementia or intellectual disability.

It seems inevitable that future developments in AI and robotics will make further inroads into health care and displace many of the functions that are currently fulfilled by human practitioners. Recently, scholars have started to speculate on how this displacement will change practice across the spectrum of the health professions.[50-57] A measure of consensus seems to be emerging that health and social care practice will change materially, with many of these changes bringing benefits to patients, clients and communities. More accurate diagnoses; improved selection of appropriate therapies for individuals; reduced complication rates from procedures; more efficient use of practitioner time; enhanced accuracy of medication prescription, dispensing and interaction checking; and improved services, especially for people who are disadvantaged or in rural and remote communities, are all postulated benefits of the technological advances to come. There seems little doubt, however, that there are some things that computers and robots will never do as well as humans, or at least not for a long time. Most authors appear to agree that the human dimensions of healthcare will remain the primary domain of the human practitioner for the foreseeable future. These include providing emotional support and compassion in times of distress; helping patients and clients to understand information about the expected effectiveness of particular treatment options and choose between them, in the light of their own circumstances and values; and ensuring that they are treated with respect for their autonomy and human dignity. Preparing learners for an increased focus on these functions will require a reprioritisation of the capabilities they will need to acquire across all three of Bloom's domains,[1] as we will discuss in Chapter 2.

4. Ready Access to 'Just-In-Time' Factual Information

Another aspect of clinical practice that has changed markedly in the last two decades follows from the advent of 'smart' devices carried in every practitioner's pocket, together with the formulation of applications and services that provide immediate access to reliable current information to inform diagnostic and treatment decisions. Examples include 'UpToDate',[58] 'Essential Evidence Plus',[59] 'DynaMed Plus'[60] and 'Epocrates'.[61] The utilisation of handheld computers in healthcare has been very well studied and, as far back as 2013, Mickan and colleagues[62] were able to bring together the findings of no less than five systematic reviews, comprising data from 138 unique primary studies. They found evidence that the use of handheld devices was associated with a range of benefits including reduced prescription error rates and 'fewer unsafe treatment decisions'[62] (p. 6). More recently, Johnson et al.[63] evaluated six of the most commonly used 'apps' for quality and ease of use. They found that they all were largely fit for purpose and found no material difference between them, despite widely differing prices. They concluded that 'selection of a mobile point-of-care tool will likely depend on individual preference'[63] (p. 6).

Fjortoft et al.[64] recently revisited the time-honoured exhortation to pharmacists-in-training to respond to questions from other health professionals or patients with 'I don't know but I can look it up and get back to you'. They note that 'looking it up' now takes only seconds and have begun to question how much health professional learners actually need to memorise in such an environment. They note that '[i]t may be more important for students to know how to quickly find and organize high quality information, and synthesize that information … to develop appropriate patient or situation specific recommendations'[64] (p. 215). Teodorczuk and colleagues[65] go even further and question whether 'in this age when practitioners have up to date knowledge at their fingertips on a device in every pocket, it might even be seen as *unprofessional*' (emphasis added) for health care workers 'to rely on fallible human memory for the recall of critical "facts" in the course of patient care'[65] (p. 529).

As Fjortoft and colleagues[64] note, these technologies are 'here to stay'[64] (p. 216) and can only be expected to improve over time. The immediate availability of reliable information at all times in practice has major implications for both goals and methods in the education and assessment of health professionals into the future. Our previous focus on 'knowledge' as a series of 'bankable' facts seems likely to need to move up the levels of Bloom and colleagues' cognitive domain.[1] In the psychomotor domain, learners will need skills in consulting the descendants of the 'apps' we have discussed in a manner that does not impair the human experience of their patients and clients during clinical encounters. As in many of the other areas discussed in this chapter, these capabilities will also need to be underpinned by the affective domain values that alert the practitioner to risks to their patients' and clients' best interests that might be introduced by the utilisation of such technologies. We will discuss the changes to our educational approaches that will be required to ensure that learners achieve these changed learning outcomes in Chapter 2.

5. Increased Reliance on Complex Technology

The need for health professionals who can not only interact with technology and informatics but also integrate those skills and understandings into their patient and client care is clear in the light of the growth of health-related technology. Patients are able to search the same sources of information consulted by their clinicians and can integrate wearable devices into their daily life. The challenge will be training healthcare professionals who can navigate all of these sources of information, drive the development of new technology and improve health outcomes for their patients. As an example, as far back as 1998, Monane et al.[66] utilised a computerised drug utilisation review system to bridge the gap between physicians, pharmacists and patients and improve suboptimal medication use. This required the collaboration of pharmacy, medicine and nursing practitioners, as well as computer programmers, to develop criteria for the system.

Over 30 years ago, the Association for American Medical Colleges first called for the inclusion of informatics in medical education.[67] Through the 1990s, physicians were dabbling in the use of computers as an adjunct to clinical decisions.[68] However, as Caroline Morton and colleagues[69] have recently observed, today there is still 'a need to train a cohort of doctors who can both practice medicine and engage in the development of useful, innovative technologies to increase efficiency and adapt to the modern medical world'[69] (para. 1).

One of the greatest challenges is to translate data into useable information. The volume of available data is exploding, as illustrated by the observation that YouTube users upload 48 hours of video and WordPress users publish 347 new log posts every minute of every day.[70] Futurists Susskind and Susskind[71] have predicted that 'machines and systems will work alongside tomorrow's professionals as partners' and argue that the challenge will be 'to allocate tasks ... according to their relative strengths'. They point out that '[h]uman professionals will have to come to terms with the need to defer to the superior capabilities of machines'[71] (p. 117).

In the last decade or so, writers from health professions as diverse as medicine,[72–74] nursing,[75] social work,[76] pharmacy[77] and psychology[78] have expressed the need for clinicians with computer coding skills. In 2011, clinical informatics became a recognised medical subspecialty in the United States.[79] The programme requirements for fellowship education in the subspecialty stipulate that clinical informaticians need to be able to analyse, implement and evaluate information and systems to improve health outcomes and strengthen the clinician–patient relationship.[80] Although the core content is comprehensive, it is primarily focused on cognitive understandings and psychomotor skills with very little attention given to learning in the affective domain.

Clearly, some health professionals will continue to specialise in this area but, as AI and robotics assume ever larger roles in healthcare and health promotion, there is an open question about whether all health professionals will ultimately need computer-coding capabilities. We would suggest the idea of 'information technology literacy' as a description for the degree to which health workers will need to understand what is going on 'under the hood' of the applications and systems they employ in order to retain professional responsibility for their practice. Such literacy would also enable health professionals to influence the ongoing development of programs and devices, and remain aware of where such developments may be covertly serving the interests of other parties in ways that might compromise the interests of their patients and clients.

As clinicians integrate informatics into health systems there must be a conscious decision to emphasise the clinician–patient relationship and a commitment to ensure that the practice of clinical informatics includes attention to the affective domain values that underpin good healthcare.

Practice Highlights

- A number of important trends in the provision of health and social care and prevention practice can be identified, including:
  1. Increasing complexity and chronicity of the world's most significant health challenges and increased recognition of the importance of the social and environmental determinants of health
  2. Increasing concern about distress and even suicide among health practitioners
  3. Developments in AI and robotics
  4. Ready access to reliable, 'just-in-time', factual information on handheld devices in the course of health practice
  5. Increased reliance on complex technology in the practice of health and social care.
- Each of these trends has implications for the education of health practitioners, across all three domains of learning: cognitive, psychomotor and affective.

Chapter 2: What?

In Chapter 1, we explored some of the emerging problems and dilemmas in health and social care practice that we can see currently or anticipate for the times ahead, as well as their implications for health professional education. In this chapter, we will consider what new educational approaches will need to be developed and what modifications of our existing practices will be required order to address the implications of these contextual changes for each of the numbered areas of expected practice change discussed in Chapter 1.

1. Interprofessional Education

We alluded in Chapter 1 to the increasing need for health professionals to acquire the capabilities required for effective interprofessional collaborative practice, across all three of

Bloom's domains.[1] Over the last decade, a consensus has emerged[81,82] that the development of such collaborative capabilities can be best achieved through *interprofessional education*. In this pedagogical approach, students or practitioners from different health professions learn 'with, from and about' each other through specifically designed learning activities (Centre for the Advancement of Interprofessional Education [CAIPE],[83] para. 2). The focus on all three prepositions in the widely adopted CAIPE definition of interprofessional education emphasises that merely including interprofessional understandings in the curriculum for health students, or even putting learners from different health professions in the same classroom to receive didactic presentations about them, are unlikely to lead to acquisition of the capabilities to which we referred in Chapter 1. The inclusion of 'from' underlines the fact that interprofessional learning activities need to involve guided interaction between students or practitioners from different professions so that they can learn about each other's expertise and perspectives.

A wide range of interprofessional learning activities has been reported over the last decade or so.[84] The majority have been undertaken during placement in real clinical settings (e.g. Wilhelmsson et al.,[85]), whereas many have been classroom-based and, more recently, a proportion have utilised simulation as the primary pedagogical methodology.[86] It has been universally recognised that the implementation of interprofessional education activities is complex and challenging, with a wide variety of obstacles identified. These include the absence of designated funding sources, 'siloed' approaches to education within each profession, the perception that curricula are 'crowded', mismatching pedagogical philosophies, limited facilitator experience of working interprofessionally and, especially, logistical problems such as location of campuses, availability of suitable teaching space, mismatches in cohort sizes and inflexibility of timetables.[87] Into the future, both organisational and technological solutions to these barriers will need to be found to facilitate the universal inclusion of interprofessional learning activities into health curricula.

As mentioned in Chapter 1, there is now a broad agreement about the capabilities that health professional students need to acquire in order to practice effectively in an interprofessional collaborative environment. Consensus has also started to emerge about how the achievement of those capabilities should be assessed. Summative assessment of interprofessional learning is seen as essential for several important reasons.[88] Firstly, assessment is vital in order to raise the value of the learning for all stakeholders and promote learner engagement in activities that may otherwise be seen as less important than disciplinary curriculum. Secondly, it serves to verify that the learner has acquired the capabilities necessary for safe and effective collaborative practice in order to meet the expectations of patients, clients and communities. Assessment also measures what learning has taken place and inspires further learning. A recent international consensus statement on the assessment of interprofessional learning outcomes[88] recommended that all pre-registration health programmes utilise at least two forms of assessment including measurement of both cognitive domain learning (through conventional tests of knowledge and understanding) and psychomotor domain interprofessional behaviour (through observation of practice either in real-care settings or in simulation). The authors of the consensus statement also recommended that further research be undertaken to identify the means through which acquisition of the affective domain values that underpin collaborative practice may be assessed.

2. Building Personal Resilience

In Chapter 1, we pointed to growing concerns about distress and even suicide among health professionals. We emphasised the importance of healthcare services making systemic change to remove avoidable sources of stress such as practitioner overwork and supervisor bullying. We also pointed out that, even in a perfect healthcare service, practice in the health professions will remain stressful because of its inherent nature. Accordingly, we concluded that developing the capability to respond to unavoidably stressful situations adaptively is critically important for health professional students.

Concerns about distress might lead to the notion that we need to revise our educational approaches in order to make them less stressful for health professional students.[89] Such an approach would, however, encompass only part of the problem. It is certainly true that we should look for sources of unnecessary and unhelpful stress in our educational and assessment practices, as well as ensuring that learners feel able to speak up about mental health concerns and access appropriate support to manage them.[90] It would, however, be naïve to believe that we could, or indeed should, eliminate stress from health professional education entirely. On the contrary, given the inherent nature of many of the sources of stress in practice, it could be argued that it is the *duty* of health professional programmes to provide opportunities to experience and manage stress during training but to do so in a carefully controlled, deliberate and considered way.

Such an approach would build on decades of experience in the use of exposure to stressful stimuli in the psychotherapeutic management of anxiety symptoms in individuals.[91] Similar strategies, described as 'stress inoculation', have also been used in the preparation of military personnel for the stress of their work[92,93] and, in a single early report, in the training of nurses.[94]

Chan and colleagues,[95] from the first author's former team, have proposed an educational model, based on the theory of contemplative pedagogy,[96] which utilises

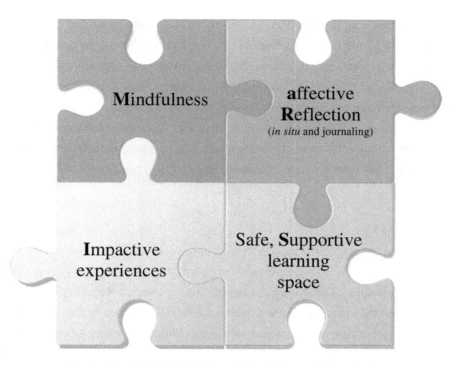

Fig. 1.   The MaRIS Model (adapted from Chan et al., 2019 [95]).

controlled graded exposure to deliberately stressful learning experiences to build both personal resilience and human capabilities in health professional learners. Their approach is known as MaRIS and combines **M**indfulness, **a**ffective **R**eflection, emotionally **I**mpactive learning experiences and a **S**upportive learning environment to these ends (see Figure 1). We will explore 'how' this model is implemented, as well potential future extensions of its use, in Chapter 3.

3. New and Reprioritised Professional Capabilities

In Chapter 1, we considered the likely increasing prominence of AI and robotics in health professional practice into the future. This anticipated practice change will require substantial reprioritisation of the capabilities that health professionals of the future will need to acquire in order to continue to add value in terms of the welfare of patients and clients in a radically changed healthcare and health promotion environment. As Susskind and Susskind[71] observed in 2015, this poses a challenge 'to allocate tasks, as between human beings and machines, according to their relative strengths' (p. 117). There is no doubt that health professional education programmes will need to take account of this challenge and redesign their curricula accordingly. There will need to be a shift of focus in the direction of the particular capabilities in which AI systems and robots will *not* surpass their human counterparts, at least not for a long time.

First among these reprioritised capabilities is likely to be, obviously enough, what Chan et al.[95] have termed 'human capabilities'. This term encompasses a cluster of learning outcomes, across all three domains of Bloom's taxonomy,[1] that are essential not only for effective interaction between health professionals (as discussed in Part 1) but also for successful engagement with patients and clients that optimises their health outcomes and their experience of the clinical encounter. Specifically, in the cognitive domain, they include an understanding of what is known about effective interpersonal communication and how it may be optimised, as well as how health information is traditionally organised into a 'history' that can facilitate the diagnostic process (increasingly with support from AI systems) and elicit the key parameters that will guide subsequent therapeutic decisions. In the psychomotor domain, human capabilities encompass conventionally-trainable 'communication skills', such as active listening, attention to body language and eye contact, as well as the appropriate use of 'minimal encouragers' to aid the patient or client's provision of additional information. Finally, in the affective domain, the acquisition of human capabilities includes alignment with the values that underpin the professional practice of the health professions and drive the behaviour that society expects of practitioners under the 'social contract'.[19]

In addition to the explicitly human capabilities just described, Wartman and Combs[97] have suggested some associated functions in relation to which humans are likely to outperform electronic systems and devices, at least for the medium term. They argue for the importance of a greater understanding of mathematics, and particularly 'sophistication in stochastic processes'[97] (p. 147), which would span both the cognitive and psychomotor domains. These capabilities are seen as necessary in order for future practitioners to be able to interpret the probabilistic outputs of AI programs meaningfully with their patients and clients. They will be rendered even more crucial by a shift towards 'personalised medicine', where the most appropriate treatments are chosen according to particular patient or client characteristics (including genetics) rather than being based on their effectiveness for the 'average' human. Here too, intellectual and procedural capabilities will need to be underpinned by learning in the affective domain that emphasises the welfare and autonomy of the patient or client over the interests of the practitioner or any commercial entities involved in the process. These interests would also need to be balanced against cost concerns and interests of the broader community, as well as of the physical environment that sustains it. As Wartman and Combs[97] point out, '[t]he ability to interpret these probabilities clearly and sensitively to patients and their families represents an additional — and essential — educational demand that speaks to a vital human, clinical, and ethical need that no amount of computing power can meet' (p. 148).

Wartman and Combs,[97] drawing on the earlier work of Tversky and Kahneman,[98] also point to the need for capabilities related to the 'psychology of choice' (p. 148) and the heuristics that humans employ in decision-making. They highlight as an example the 'framing effect' in decision-making about serious matters that can lead to 'evidence of harm' being perceived by patients and clients as 'more compelling than evidence of effectiveness'[98] (p. 148). In the light of this, if the affectively learned ethical principle of beneficence is to be upheld and balanced against respect for autonomy in helping patients and clients make difficult personal treatment choices, health workers will also need a cognitive understanding of these phenomena and (psychomotor domain) practice at utilising them in clinical consultation.

4. Authentic Assessment of Learning Outcomes

In Chapter 1, we considered the educational implications of the immediate availability, in the present and into the future, of relevant and reliable factual information to guide patient and client care via a 'smart' device in every practitioner's pocket. In this environment, our erstwhile focus on health professional students acquiring the 'knowledge' required for future practice needs to be re-examined. Outcomes at the lower levels of Bloom and colleagues' cognitive domain,[1] with initial verbs like 'name', 'describe' or 'discuss', have been the mainstay of health professional learning descriptions since the move towards defining clear objectives or outcomes began in the 1950s and 1960s. When these kinds of outcomes can be met in seconds with a few swipes and clicks on a device, there seems little point in asking our present and future students to spend their time learning to meet them. Accordingly, our outcome descriptions will need to move up Bloom's levels to focus on higher order learning with verbs like 'apply', 'employ', 'analyse', 'criticise', 'synthesise' and 'appraise'.

Promoting higher order cognitive learning outcomes has, of course, been the stated intention of health professional educators since at least the 1970s when problem-based learning (PBL) approaches began to be disseminated from their origins at McMaster Medical School.[99] We have preached this to our students and, over the last few years in particular, bemoaned their attempts to undermine our efforts through the development and inheritance between cohorts of 'supernotes' for each of our PBL cases.[65] What we don't often appreciate is that the reason that our students see activities like PBL (without 'supernotes') as 'low yield' is that we still assess them in a manner that rewards memorisation of 'facts' over higher order learning outcomes.

The assessment of cognitive learning in most health professional programmes utilises a combination of single best answer multiple choice questions and short answer questions based on clinical scenarios, undertaken under 'exam conditions', where candidates are required to answer entirely from their own resources and the consultation of notes or other materials is prohibited. In this modality, even if we have worked hard to write questions that require clinical reasoning and application of learnt understandings to new settings, recollection of memorised facts is still required and rewarded. As we have seen, such an assessment environment is utterly different from real healthcare practice in the present and the future. In the real world, practitioners now have immediate access to any facts that they need to perform their role and, as we discussed in Chapter 1, should actually be discouraged from reliance on fallible 'wetware' for critical information.

This changed environment demands a radical change in our assessment methodologies. Teodorczuk and colleagues[65] have suggested that the introduction of open-book examinations — which have a long history in legal education[100] — may provide a more authentic form of assessment that will discourage memorisation and promote higher order learning. They suggest that this approach might also reduce the stress that learners experience in preparing for exams. In addition, they argue that allowing candidates access to information materials during assessment may even provide a solution to the often-cited problem of the 'crowded curriculum', since this concern is predicated on a view of curriculum as a large number of (lower order) things to be learnt.

For these reasons, open-book written exams certainly appear to warrant further investigation. However, the assessment of cognitive learning outcomes is not the only area where access to information sources would enhance assessment authenticity. The prohibition of such access during clinical assessments such as Observed Structured Clinical Examinations,[101] long cases and mini-clinical evaluation exercises (CEXs)[102] also makes little sense if we really wish to determine whether candidates have the capabilities to undertake their professional duties as they are actually practised in contemporary times. Indeed, psychomotor domain, trainable, skills in utilising point-of-care information apps, as well as the affective domain values that underpin them, will themselves need to be assessed if we are to verify that our graduates are truly ready for practice in today's and tomorrow's clinical world.

In Chapter 3, we will consider how emerging technologies may help to overcome the difficulties inherent in assessing health students authentically into the future.

5. Information Technological Literacy

In Chapter 1, we pointed to the importance of ensuring that health professionals of the future are information technology literate so that they can fulfil their professional responsibilities when utilising new technologies in healthcare and health promotion. Incorporating informatics and technology literacy into health professional education requires institutional commitment. Kotter's eight steps for institutional change[103] delineate a series of phases that, he observes, can take considerable time and effort to be successful. Professional education programmes that do not currently include informatics and technology literacy content need to adopt a sense of urgency, Kotter's first step. Wartman[104] has noted that '[i]t should be evident that the accelerating pace of change in medicine and health care directly impacts universities' health entities' (para. 7). He suggests that '[t]o adapt — and indeed thrive — these institutions need to develop a strong culture of innovation and experimentation' noting that this will be challenging in the face of an existing 'culture of academic individualism and entrenched programs and policies'. Wartman goes on to argue that '[c]reating a "frictionless environment" for experimentation in partnership with the tech sector is a tall but necessary order as the coming environment requires lowering the barriers to innovation'[104] (para. 7).

As we consider technology literacy education, computer science pedagogy is a field that may assist in providing model practices for educating health professionals. Researchers in Spain[105] created a series of computer programming learning tools explicitly based upon Bloom's taxonomy.[1] The learning tools were developed to progress a student through the levels of the taxonomy's cognitive domain. Other scholars[106] have suggested, however, that the *synthesis* and *evaluation* levels of Bloom's taxonomy may not be appropriate to computer science education. This was taken a step further with a cluster analysis study of programming students, which found that even though some students performed poorly on 'lower' levels of the taxonomy, they still performed well at 'higher' levels.[107] Fuller's group[108] has proposed a new taxonomy adapted from Bloom's structure. All of this work has focused particularly on the cognitive domain, but it is clear that the other two domains of Bloom's taxonomy will also be important when informatics is incorporated into health professional education. The affective domain will be particularly pertinent, as learners will need to base their health informatics practice on application of the values that underpin their professions, particularly integrity and placing the interests of patients and clients first.[109] Technological learning for health professionals is also likely to include learning new psychomotor skills for interacting with systems that are second nature to computer scientists but unfamiliar to learners from other fields. In relation to health professional education, Shortliffe[110] has argued that '[b]iomedical informatics is not a topic that is optimally taught in a single course during the preclinical years but rather should be blended into the … curriculum with evolving topics and the use of clinical examples and challenges to motivate and direct the grasp of informatics concepts' (p. 1228).

A number of examples of the integration of information technology literacy into medical education have been reported over the last decade. An undergraduate medical programme in

Mexico developed a two-semester informatics course sequence that focused on core concepts (in the cognitive domain) and the processes of decision-making and clinical reasoning (arguably in the psychomotor domain), but with little attention to affective domain learning.[111] They reported that their blended-learning education model was well received by students and teachers but required local 'champions' who could supplement the institution's faculty in teaching the new content.

Researchers in the United Kingdom studied the efficacy of a two-day course on computer programming for a group of undergraduate medical students.[69] The course was designed to develop basic programme-writing skills, the ability to discuss computational thinking and projects with computer scientists. This would appear to be close to the concept of 'information technology literacy' that we suggested in Chapter 1. They found that students were able to create simple but useful clinical programmes. This learning activity focused on cognitive understanding and psychomotor domain skills but, again, there was no discussion of the affective domain dimensions of the use of information technology in healthcare.

In China, Teng and Wang[112] studied how to improve learning in a pathology course by integrating information literacy content. They utilised a pathology cases database, digital sections library and a blog-based teaching platform to deliver content and assess student learning. Their description appears to have focused on the lower levels of the cognitive domain.

On a grander scale, Silverman et al.[113] reported the development of a new medical school curriculum that incorporated over 45 hours of required, sequenced and integrated informatics instruction across the 4-year curriculum. Self-assessment rating scores by students indicated improved understanding and acceptance of technology and its role in patient care. The self-assessment was focused on cognitive and some affective domain outcomes, but these scholars do not appear to have assessed psychomotor skills.

As we can see from these examples, a variety of approaches is being adopted to attempt to integrate information technology literacy into medical education. Some programmes focus on cognitive knowledge concerning technology systems whereas others incorporate the psychomotor skills of actual programming. It is important to note that no single method will be effective across international and cultural boundaries. Each institution will need to balance facilities, resources, faculty expertise and student prior knowledge. It can be anticipated that future generations of students, who have grown up immersed in technology, may come into programmes with higher levels of literacy and prerequisite knowledge. The assumption that members of the so-called 'Generation Y' were 'digital natives' has been questioned,[114] but their successors will be learning computer coding compulsorily at primary school, at least in some parts of the world,[115] and the challenge may be finding faculty who can keep up with the students.

Practice Highlights

- Each of the trends in health and social care practice identified in Chapter 1 requires new or revised approaches to health professional education, across the three domains of learning, as follows:
  1. Interprofessional education to develop the collaborative practice capabilities that health practitioners will require, to address the increasing complexity and chronicity of their work, as well as the social and environmental determinants of health, into the future
  2. Approaches that are effective in building the personal resilience needed to manage the unavoidable stresses of health practice
  3. New and reprioritised professional capabilities as many traditional tasks of health practice are delegated to AI systems and robots
  4. Authentic assessment of learning outcomes in a changed environment where reliance on human memory for critical information is arguably unprofessional
  5. Development of information technology literacy to enable practitioners to fulfil their professional duties to ensure patient and client welfare when complex AI systems and robots are being deployed in health practice.

Chapter 3: How?

In Chapter 1 of this section, we discussed what we see as emerging problems in health and social care practice and anticipated what further changes we may see in the field in the years ahead. We also explored the implications of these concerns and likely changes for health professional educators. In Chapter 2, we examined what modifications of our educational practices, as well as what new approaches, may need to be developed in order to respond to this changing landscape. In this chapter, we will explore emerging and anticipated educational methodologies that might enable us to implement these new and modified approaches.

1. 'Second Generation' Interprofessional Education

In Chapters 1 and 2, we explored the growing need for health practitioners to acquire the capabilities required to work together effectively across professional boundaries in order to prevent and manage the increasingly complex and chronic health problems that face diverse communities with aging population profiles. We described the range of interprofessional learning activities that have been trialled to date and the barriers to their implementation.

We also looked specifically at why and how the acquisition of interprofessional capabilities can be assessed.

As we have discussed, interprofessional education is difficult to do, but there is the potential for both organisational and technological innovations to render its effective implementation more achievable. In the organisational sphere, among the greatest challenges is achieving ongoing collaboration and coordination between teachers in different health professional disciplines in order to sustain interprofessional learning activities in the face of staff changes, timetable revisions and modifications to individual programmes over time. Teodorczuk et al.[18] have suggested the formation of a regularly meeting steering group comprising a mix of official representatives from each school or department (with the *imprimatur* to make decisions), together with interprofessional education 'champions' to provide the enthusiasm and connection to purpose that are vital to maintain the effort over the long term.

Another organisational innovation that might support learners' acquisition of collaborative capabilities is a *programmatic* approach to interprofessional education.[116] Under this model, learning from the most intensive, fully interactive interprofessional activities can be augmented by the utilisation of simpler activities earlier and later in each student's programme of study. Activities would be matched to the learner's stage of professional development in a purposive way. For example, students will gain much more from a high-cost, organisationally demanding, simulated interprofessional team experience around the middle of their pre-registration programmes if they have previously undertaken more conventional learning activities to build their understanding of the various health professions and their roles, as well as what is known about effective interprofessional communication, in the cognitive domain. Similarly, a programmatic approach allows for the utilisation of 'capstone' activities towards the end of students' programmes where, for example, they are asked to critique the interprofessional functioning of a real health team that they have had the opportunity to observe during clinical placement. Such activities have the potential to reactivate, enhance and operationalise the interprofessional learning acquired across a structured programme and, in doing so, may serve to 'immunise' graduates against enculturation to suboptimal collaborative practice environments after graduation.[116]

Extended live action simulations of subsequent professional life have been shown to be effective in ensuring the acquisition of professional and interprofessional capabilities across all three of Bloom's domains of learning.[1,117,118] Virtual reality technologies may have the potential to produce similar results into the future while enabling learners to experience collaborative simulations without needing to be geographically co-located. There have been a couple of reports to date of the use of the virtual simulated environment known as Second

Life for interprofessional education, e.g.,[119,120] but, so far, the fidelity of available technologies limits the quality of the learning, especially in the psychomotor and affective domains. Once technology of the kind imagined in the *Star Trek* 'holodeck'[121] becomes available, this may become the primary mode for experiential learning across the health professions but this degree of realism is probably a long way in the future. In the meantime, 'augmented reality', which 'supplements the real world with virtual objects, such that virtual objects appear to coexist in the same space as the real world'[122] (p. 1) may be a better prospect for adding to the learning effectiveness of live action simulations.

The kind of hybrid simulation described in our scenario, where learners from different professions work with live SPs to learn the more human dimensions of their work while virtual characters and objects are added to display particular pathologies, is probably not all that far off. Fulfilling the goal of enabling students from different geographical locations to learn with and learn from each other through the use of AR — in the manner imagined in meetings of the Jedi High Council in the *Star Wars* film series[123] — would also not require much further development of currently available technologies.

In our scenario, the AR interprofessional learning activities in which Yu Yan was participating had been designed and kept current by a steering group formulated and sustained according to Teodorczuk and colleagues'[18] recommendations, as part of a carefully structured sequence of interprofessional learning activities and assessments across the length of her university programme. The utilisation of both the organisational and technological innovations we have described might become known as 'second generation' interprofessional education.

2. New Ways to Build Human Capabilities and Personal Resilience in Practitioners

In Chapters 1 and 2 of this section, we discussed the adverse consequences for health professionals, as well as their patients and clients, of the stresses that are experienced in practice. We also pointed to the potential for controlled and graded exposure to deliberately designed emotionally impactive learning experiences, in a supportive environment, to build both personal resilience and human capabilities among health professional students.

Under the MaRIS model, which we introduced in Chapter 2,[95] learners work in groups of six, each with an expert facilitator and undertake multiple workshops over a period of several weeks. Each session begins with a secular mindfulness meditation exercise to assist students to clear their minds and focus on the learning activity.[124] The facilitator assists participants to translate the experience of this exercise to create a mindful approach to the entirety of the workshop and indeed to all of their learning in classroom, simulation and real care settings into the future. Once a mindful tone has been established, participants review together the content of workshop, which has been introduced in a large group learning session a few days before. Then, each member of the group, in turn, undertakes a simulated consultation encounter with a different human SP who has been specially trained to perform the role of a particular patient or client authentically. Early in the programme of workshops, students are asked to undertake relatively straightforward clinical interactions, such as assisting the patient or client to provide a history of their presenting problem. At the beginning, inexperienced learners find even these fairly simple encounters to be quite emotionally impactive.

After each encounter, the student first describes the experience of the activity to their colleagues, reflects aloud on its meaning and critiques their own performance. Then, the SP (who has 'broken character' at this point) provides feedback on how the learner came across on a human level, before leaving the room to 'rotate' to the next student group and perform the same role for a different learner. The other participants in the group then provide feedback on both the content and human dimensions of the consultation and, finally, the facilitator sums up the feedback and provides their own. The next student in the group then invites in a new SP, playing a different character, and the process is repeated. Across the course of the workshops, the learners are guided by the facilitator to provide their feedback in a constructive and collegial manner, ensuring that the mindful and supportive environment of the workshop is maintained.

The final component of the MaRIS model is affective reflection. During the workshop, learners are encouraged by their facilitators to focus on their feelings during each encounter and also how they can make sense of what they have experienced to better understand themselves *vis-à-vis* their future practice as health professionals. This live reflection is augmented by requiring the students also to reflect in writing about their overall experience of several of the workshops and the activities' impact on their developing professional identity. These writings are summatively assessed to encourage student engagement, utilising a specially developed methodology[118] and tool[125] designed to identify to presence and quality of affective learning evidenced. Learners are also provided with feedback on their journals to build their capability in affective reflection over time.

Chan and colleagues[95] have shown that across a series of MaRIS-based workshops, learners' self-assessed empathy, resilience and sense of human capability steadily increase. As learners progress through the programme, the complexity and sensitivity of the SP encounters is increased, with the incorporation of scenarios such as sexual health histories or 'breaking bad news'. This sustains their emotional impactiveness in the face of increasing learner confidence and so further builds their personal resilience and human capabilities.

Wider implementation of this model into the future, integrated, where appropriate, with the AR and AI elements discussed above, can be expected to impact positively on graduates' ability to respond adaptively to the stresses inherent in health professional practice. It will also build the human capabilities and tolerance of uncertainty they will require to engage effectively with the increasingly complex health problems they can be expected to encounter.

3. Innovations to Enable Acquisition of New and Reprioritised Capabilities

In Chapter 1, we considered the impact of the increasing utilisation of AI and robotics on the daily work of human health professionals into the future. In Chapter 2, we identified a resultant range of new and reprioritised capabilities that health graduates will require in order to continue to contribute usefully to the welfare of patients, clients and communities in the world ahead. In this chapter, we will consider how these capabilities might best be acquired in the health professional school of 2030.

As we alluded to in the original scenario and the earlier parts of this chapter, simulation is already a vital tool in the armamentarium of the health professional educator and further advances in simulation practice and technology offer exciting prospects for the future. In the first part, we pointed to the utility of extended multi-method simulations of junior practitioner life specifically to develop health students' interprofessional collaborative practice capabilities.[18,117,118] Similarly, these methodologies have proven useful in building the broader set of 'human capabilities',[95,118] the application of which will become an ever-greater part of health professionals' work as AI and robotics displace humans from the tasks that the machines will perform more effectively. The addition of virtual and, especially, AR components to extended simulations that also include human SPs and mechanical mannequin simulators has the potential to further advance this aim.

In the Clinical Learning through Extended Immersion in Multi-method Simulation (CLEIMS) methodology,[18,117,118] educators from Griffith University in Australia have utilised a seamless combination of live SP scenarios (including the patients' significant others) and mannequin-based simulation to create week-long realistic simulations of the practice of an interprofessional healthcare team. These include the simulated ordering and receipt of investigations in real time; the necessity to undertake diagnostic formulation 'on the fly'; counselling of patients and their relatives, with shared decision-making; and low-tech online after hours 'ward call' tasks, to create an authentic experience of junior practitioner life. Published evaluations have shown sustained educational value across all three of Bloom and colleagues'[1] domains of learning.[117,118] It is easy to imagine (as we have in our initial scenario) how the addition of AR components to a CLEIMS-like extended simulation, through the use of wearable devices descended from 'Google Glass',[126] might enable ever-more complex and realistic simulations of practice. These could overlay simulated injuries and physical signs onto the bodies of live SPs and clients, or onto mannequins where appropriate, to create clinical experiences that are difficult to simulate with present technology. The presence of live simulation performers will remain important to the development of human capabilities however, at least for the medium term, as it is unlikely that computerised simulations of patients and clients will be sufficiently accurate to evoke the authentic emotional responses that are critical to affective learning.[95,118]

In this kind of learning environment, it would be relatively easy to create elements within the extended scenario that require health professional learners to synthesise the available information, apply the mathematical capabilities and decision psychology understandings alluded to in Chapter 2[97] and then assist patients and clients to make treatment decisions that accord with their personal values and desired outcomes. The utilisation of affective reflection, as discussed in Part 2 of this chapter, in association with these impactive simulated learning experiences, will assist students to acquire (and educators to verify the acquisition of) the affective domain learning that will underpin their ongoing practice in this changed environment.

4. Enhanced Assessment Methodologies

In Chapter 1, we observed that ready access to reliable information to guide diagnostic and treatment decisions via handheld devices is already usual practice in the health professions. We noted that this phenomenon appeared to be preferable to reliance on fallible human memory for critical information and thus should enhance patient and client safety. Equally, such point-of-care information applications could be regularly updated and accessed more efficiently than similar materials in printed form. In Chapter 2, we argued that the availability of immediate access to factual information in all practice settings into the future fundamentally changes the nature of health professional education. It enables learners to move away from a focus on the mere acquisition of professional knowledge towards achievement of higher order learning outcomes, especially in the cognitive domain. We went on to suggest that our assessment methodologies had not yet recognised these changes in clinical practice in their continued requirement for, and rewarding of, the memorisation of facts.

In Chapter 2, we suggested that allowing access to sources of information that are now readily available to practising clinicians would improve the authenticity of assessments in health professional programmes. Teodorczuk and colleagues[65] have suggested the term 'open resource' (rather than 'open book') as a more contemporary description of such examinations, with the hope that their implementation might result in learners prioritising their learning time 'away from libraries and towards the rich, but messy, clinical learning environments' (pp. 529–530). They also point to a dilemma inherent in allowing access to the internet during examinations, noting that such access 'might give rise to concerns about undetected collaboration between candidates or with others "on the outside" during assessments'[65] (p. 530). This is indeed an important problem because — although consulting with colleagues is also an aspect of real healthcare practice — educational institutions have an important requirement to verify the capability of each individual candidate in order to determine whether they are progressing appropriately, and are ultimately safe to enter professional practice.

Another dimension of our current assessment methodologies that is clearly no longer fit for purpose is the requirement that candidates write their responses to short answer questions by hand. The use of handwriting appears be becoming rare in both health professional practice and health professional education. More than 99% of Australian general medical practices are now computerised[127] and the roll-out of electronic medical records in hospitals is also well underway. The most recent study of computer use by medical students we could find[128] showed that in Iran at that time 100% of learners had access to a computer and 97% utilised one at university. Based on this, it seems likely — and accords with our informal observations — that by the present time almost all health students in developed countries are using electronic devices as their primary means of study-related writing. There is also evidence that the regular use of electronic means for creation of text leads to reduced capacity to perform the physical act of writing by hand effectively and comfortably, especially for prolonged periods.[129] Accordingly, it is becoming increasingly unreasonable and inauthentic to expect that health students will be able to hand-write answers in high stakes assessments.

Interestingly, new technologies are already emerging that may allow electronic text entry and access to online resources during assessment, replicating the context of real clinical practice, but simultaneously prevent candidates from communicating with each other or with confederates outside the assessment room. 'ExamSoft' proprietary software[130] already allows for assessments to be downloaded to users' devices in encrypted form and then activated when the exam begins, 'locking down' the device from access to other programs or the internet during the assessment and then 'sealing' and re-encrypting the responses at the end of the exam for later submission. A nationally funded Australian higher education project[131] has recently demonstrated similar capabilities with open-source software and has also trialled the use of 'whitelisting' of acceptable internet sites and logging of all candidate online activity during exams. This work seems likely to result, very soon, in a workable capability for 'open resource' assessments to be offered with electronic text entry and prevention, or at least detection, of unwanted collusion.

Similarly, it would be easy to translate more authentic assessment approaches into the verification of clinical competence. It would be a simple step to allow candidates access to whatever mobile applications they normally use during all clinical assessments and, indeed, specific practical assessments could be devised to verify their psychomotor domain capabilities in deploying such tools effectively and in a patient- and client-friendly manner in simulated clinical settings. An early forerunner of this kind of assessment was the development of an Observed Structured Clinical Examination (OSCE) station on 'evidence-based medicine' where candidates were required to research the answer to a particular clinical question 'live' in front of an examiner.[132] As technological and simulation capabilities improve, as discussed earlier in this chapter, it appears likely that ever more accurate simulations of authentic clinical practice will be utilised for assessment as well as learning purposes.

The assessment of learning in the affective domain will also be increasingly important in order to verify that health practitioners have acquired the professional values to ensure that the best interests of their patients and clients are protected in the increasing complex technological world of the future. The methodology for measuring the presence and quality of affective learning in the textual reflective journals of health students,[118,125] referred to in Part 2 of this chapter, has been shown to be sufficiently robust and reliable for medium stakes summative purposes. Into the future it is likely that this kind of approach will need to be applied to other forms of learner reflection such as the video journal that Yu Yan completed in our original scenario.

5. Gaining Information Technology Literacy

In Chapters 2 and 3, we suggested that in order for health practitioners of the future to fulfil their professional responsibilities they will need to acquire a measure of information technology literacy. They will require sufficient understanding of the ways that new applications and devices used in health practice actually work (in the cognitive domain of learning) in order to verify that they are being used appropriately, and for their patients' and clients' genuine benefit rather than primarily serving the interests of third parties. Practitioners will need trainable skills (in the psychomotor domain) in order to be able to contribute to the ongoing development of these innovations, to explain the meaning of their outputs for individual patients and clients, and to engage in collaborative decision-making with them on this basis. They will also need affective domain learning to acquire the values that the community expects of health professionals, under the social contract,[19] and be able to apply them in this brave new world. Ongoing increases in the complexity of health professional practice, in the face of developing technology, will also mandate that the assessment of competence be a life-long process that, when done carefully, can provide insight into performance, generate new knowledge and increase the capacity to adapt to change.[133]

For this final part, we will revisit our initial scenario to look at how the development of information technology literacy may be added seamlessly to the future health professional pedagogies we have imagined. As we saw at the beginning of the section, Yu Yan was undertaking an interprofessional learning programme that challenged her and her colleagues to interact with, assess, diagnose and treat a mixture of live SPs and AR avatars with a range of problems.

At several points in this activity, she might be presented with instances where slavishly following the recommendations of an AI application that she consults will **not** actually be in her patient's best interests and may pose a risk of harm. In one example, the algorithm might have failed to ask for or take account of an individual characteristic of her patient (such as a co-morbidity, another medication the patient is taking or a known genetic variation) that is critical to the decision-making. At this point, she would be assessed on her ability to look 'under the hood' to determine how the code was written and the data aggregated. She will need to consult her informatics instructor (who may be a live human at a remote location or even another avatar) and work with the specialist to modify the application to mitigate its newly discovered deficiency.

In another case, the AI system consulted might be deliberately programmed to recommend a particular brand of drug over cheaper, but equally effective, alternatives because the system was developed by the (fictitious) pharmaceutical company that stands to benefit. The capability under assessment here will be a critical sensitivity to whose interest is being served when technological aids are developed and offered for clinical use. The assessment process would include analysis of her video journal about what she has learned from this experience in the affective domain and how this deeper understanding about the risks that vested interests may pose to patient and client welfare is incorporated into future practice.

Practice Highlights

- Innovative learning methodologies will be required to allow implementation of the new and reprioritised learning approaches identified in Chapter 3. These include:
  1. 'Second generation' interprofessional education utilising enhanced simulation and a programmatic approach
  2. The utilisation of new ways to build human capabilities and personal resilience in practitioners, incorporating mindfulness, affective reflection and emotionally impactive learning experiences in a supportive environment, based on the MaRIS model

3. Innovations to enable acquisition of new and reprioritised capabilities in the face of displacement of tasks to AI and robots, such as extended interprofessional clinical simulations, supported by human patient simulation and AR devices

4. Enhanced assessment methodologies that take account of the shift to higher order learning outcomes as the immediate availability of accurate information obviates the need for memorisation

5. New methodologies to enable health students to gain information technology literacy.

References

1. Bloom BS, Engelhart MD, Furst EJ, Hill WH, Krahwohl DR. *Taxonomy of Educational Objectives. Vol. 1: Cognitive Domain*. New York: McKay; 1956:7–8.

2. United Nations DESA, Population Division. *World Population Prospects: The 2017 Revision, Key Findings and Advance Tables*. New York: United Nations DESA; 2017.

3. Harrison C, Henderson J, Miller G, Britt H. The prevalence of complex multimorbidity in Australia. *Australian and New Zealand Journal of Public Health*. 2016;40(3):239–44.

4. Buttorff C, Ruder T, Bauman M. *Multiple Chronic Conditions in the United States*. Santa Monica: RAND Corporation; 2017. Available from: https://www.rand.org/content/dam/rand/pubs/tools/TL200/TL221/RAND_TL221.pdf.

5. Picco L, Achilla E, Abdin E, Chong SA, Vaingankar JA, McCrone P, et al. Economic burden of multimorbidity among older adults: Impact on healthcare and societal costs. *BMC Health Services Research*. 2016;16:173.

6. Braillard O, Slama-Chaudhry A, Joly C, Perone N, Beran D. The impact of chronic disease management on primary care doctors in Switzerland: A qualitative study. *BMC Family Practice*. 2018;19(1):159.

7. Clark NM, Gong M. Management of chronic disease by practitioners and patients: are we teaching the wrong things? *BMJ* (*Clinical Research Ed.*). 2000;320(7234):572–5.

8. Black D, Morris J, Smith C, Townsend P. Report of the working group on inequalities in Health, 1980. In: P. Townsend ND, M. Whiteheads, editors. *Inequalities in Health*. London: Penguin Books; 1988.

9. Rose G, Marmot MG. Social class and coronary heart disease. *British Heart Journal*. 1981;45(1):13–9.

10. Krieger N. Epidemiology and the People's Health: Theory and Context. New York: Oxford University Press; 2011.

11. World Health Organisation. *Closing the Gap: Policy into Practice on Social Determinants of Health: Discussion Paper*. Geneva: World Health Organisation; 2011.

12. Watts N, Amann M, Ayeb-Karlsson S, Belesova K, Bouley T, Boykoff M, et al. The Lancet Countdown on health and climate change: From 25 years of inaction to a global transformation for public health. *The Lancet*. 2018;391(10120):581–630.

13. Baines R, Langelaan M, de Bruijne M, Spreeuwenberg P, Wagner C. How effective are patient safety initiatives? A retrospective patient record review study of changes to patient safety over time. *BMJ Quality & Safety*. 2015;24(9):561–71.

14. British Royal Infirmary Inquiry. *Learning from Bristol: The Report of the Public Inquiry into Childrens Heart Surgery at the Bristol Royal Infirmary, 1984–1995*. London: The Stationery Office Books; 2001:538.

15. Garling P. *Final Report of the Special Commission of Inquiry into Acute Care Services in NSW Public Hospitals*. Sydney: New South Wales Public Hospitals; 2008.

16. Francis R. *Report of the Mid Staffordshire NHS Foundation Trust Public Inquiry*. London: The Stationery Office; 2013.

17. Rogers G, Chesters J. An orchestral metaphor for interprofessional collaborative practice? *The Clinical Teacher*. 2014;11(4):317–8.

18. Teodorczuk A, Khoo TK, Morrissey S, Rogers G. Developing interprofessional education: Putting theory into practice. *The Clinical Teacher*. 2016;13(1):7–12.

19. Cruess RL, Cruess SR, Johnston SE. Professionalism and medicine's social contract. *Journal of Bone and Joint Surgery. American Volume*. 2000;82(8):1189–94.

20. O'Keefe M, Henderson A, Chick R. Defining a set of common interprofessional learning competencies for health profession students. *Medical Teacher*. 2017;39(5):463–8.

21. Aubusson K. 'She was eaten alive': Chloe Abbott's sister Micaela's message for the next generation of doctors. *The Sydney Morning Herald*. 2017.

22. Beyond Blue. *National Mental Health Survey of Doctors and Medical Students*. Hawthorn: Beyond Blue; 2019.

23. Chang E, Eddins-Folensbee F, Coverdale J. Survey of the prevalence of burnout, stress, depression, and the use of supports by medical students at one school. *Academic Psychiatry*. 2012;36(3):177–82.

24. Dyrbye L, Shanafelt T. A narrative review on burnout experienced by medical students and residents. *Medical Education*. 2016;50(1):132–49.

25. Susan AM. Unbroken: After Dr Andrew Bryant's Suicide 2017; 17 May 2019. Available from: http://andrewmcmillen.com/2017/09/04/the-weekend-australian-magazine-story-susan-unbroken-after-dr-andrew-bryants-suicide-september-2017/.

26. Kemp S, Hu W, Bishop J, Forrest K, Hudson JN, Wilson I, et al. Medical student wellbeing — a consensus statement from Australia and New Zealand. *BMC Medical Education*. 2019;19(1):69.

27. Quine L. Workplace bullying in junior doctors: Questionnaire survey. *The BMJ*. 2002;324(7342):878–9.

28. World Medical Association. WMA Statment on Physicians Well-Being [press release]. Ferney-Voltaire: World Medical Association; 2019.

29. Boud D, Molloy E. Rethinking models of feedback for learning: the challenge of design. *Assessment & Evaluation in Higher Education*. 2013;38(6):698–712.

30. Ilgen JS, Eva KW, de Bruin A, Cook DA, Regehr G. Comfort with uncertainty: Reframing our conceptions of how clinicians navigate complex clinical situations. *Advances in Health Sciences Education. Theory and Practice*. 2019;24(4):797–809.

31. Bellolio MF, Cabrera D, Sadosty AT, Hess EP, Campbell RL, Lohse CM, et al. Compassion fatigue is similar in emergency medicine residents compared to other medical and surgical specialties. *The Western Journal of Emergency Medicine*. 2014;15(6):629–35.

32. Paro HB, Silveira PS, Perotta B, Gannam S, Enns SC, Giaxa RR, et al. Empathy among medical students: Is there a relation with quality of life and burnout? *PLoS One*. 2014;9(4):e94133.

33. Thomas MR, Dyrbye LN, Huntington JL, Lawson KL, Novotny PJ, Sloan JA, et al. How do distress and well-being relate to medical student empathy? A multicenter study. *Journal of General Internal Medicine*. 2007;22(2):177–83.

34. Ye Y, Hu R, Ni Z, Jiang N, Jiang X. Effects of perceived stress and professional values on clinical performance in practice nursing students: A structural equation modeling approach. *Nurse Education Today*. 2018;71:157–62.

35. Teodorczuk A, Thomson R, Chan K, Rogers GD. When I say ... resilience. *Medical Education*. 2017;51(12):1206–8.

36. Moor J. The Dartmouth College artificial intelligence conference: The next fifty years. *AI Magazine*. 2006;27(4):87–91.

37. René D. Discourse on the method of rightly conducting one's reason and of seeking truth in the sciences 1637; 2008. Available from: http://www.gutenberg.org/files/59/59-h/59-h.htm.

38. Kaplan A, Haenlein M. Siri, Siri, in my hand: Who's the fairest in the land? On the interpretations, illustrations, and implications of artificial intelligence. *Business Horizons*. 2019;62(1):15–25.

39. Samuel AL. Some studies in machine learning using the game of checkers. *IBM Journal of Research and Development*. 1959;3(3):210–29.

40. Dictionary OE. Robotics: Oxford English Dictionary; 2019 Available from: https://en.oxforddictionaries.com/definition/robotics.

41. Yu VL, Fagan LM, Wraith SM, Clancey WJ, Scott AC, Hannigan J, et al. Antimicrobial selection by a computer. A blinded evaluation by infectious diseases experts. *JAMA*. 1979;242(12):1279–82.

42. Gulshan V, Peng L, Coram M, Stumpe MC, Wu D, Narayanaswamy A, et al. Development and validation of a deep learning algorithm for detection of diabetic retinopathy in retinal fundus photographs. *JAMA*. 2016;316(22):2402–10.

43. Lakhani P, Sundaram B. Deep learning at chest radiography: Automated classification of pulmonary tuberculosis by using convolutional neural networks. *Radiology*. 2017;284(2):574–82.

44. Esteva A, Kuprel B, Novoa RA, Ko J, Swetter SM, Blau HM, et al. Dermatologist-level classification of skin cancer with deep neural networks. *Nature*. 2017;542(7639):115–8.

45. Asimov, I. (1969). Segregationist. In I. Asimov, *Nightfall and Other Stories* (pp 337–342). Garden City, NY: Doubleday.

46. Kwoh YS, Hou J, Jonckheere EA, Hayati S. A robot with improved absolute positioning accuracy for CT guided stereotactic brain surgery. *IEEE Transactions on Biomedical Engineering*. 1988;35(2):153–60.

47. Marino MV, Shabat G, Gulotta G, Komorowski AL. From illusion to reality: A brief history of robotic surgery. *Surgical Innovation*. 2018;25(3):291–6.

48. Soto F, Chrostowski R. Frontiers of medical micro/nanorobotics: In vivo applications and commercialization perspectives toward clinical uses. *Frontiers in Bioengineering and Biotechnology*. 2018;6:170.

49. Wilson R, Kenny C. *Robotics in Social Care.* London: The Parlimentary Office of Science and Technology; 2018.

50. Buch VH, Ahmed I, Maruthappu M. Artificial intelligence in medicine: current trends and future possibilities. *British Journal of General Practice.* 2018;68(668):143–4.

51. de Mello FL, de Souza SA. Psychotherapy and artificial intelligence: A proposal for alignment. *Frontiers in Psychology.* 2019;10:263.

52. Flynn A. Using artificial intelligence in health-system pharmacy practice: Finding new patterns that matter. *American Journal of Health-System Pharmacy.* 2019;76(9):622–7.

53. Liu L. Occupational therapy in the fourth industrial revolution. *Canadian Journal of Occupational Therapy.* 2018;85(4):272–83.

54. Pepito JA, Locsin R. Can nurses remain relevant in a technologically advanced future? *International Journal of Nursing Sciences.* 2019;6(1):106–10.

55. Tack C. Artificial intelligence and machine learning | applications in musculoskeletal physiotherapy. *Musculoskeletal Science and Practice.* 2019;39:164–9.

56. Tambe M, Rice E, (Eds.). *Artificial Intelligence and Social Work.* Cambridge: Cambridge University Press. 2018:266.

57. Zignoli A. How AI is (not) Going to Change Sport Science; 2019. Available from: https://hiitscience.com/how-ai-is-not-going-to-change-sport-science/.

58. Kluwer W. Uptodate: Wolters Kluwer; 2019. Available from: https://www.uptodate.com/home.

59. John Wiley & Sons. *Essential Evidence Plus.* John Wiley & Sons; 2019. Available from: https://www.essentialevidenceplus.com/product/.

60. Industries E. DynaMed: EBSCO Industries; 2019. Available from: https://www.dynamed.com/home.

61. Athenahealth. Epocrates: Athenahealth, Inc.; 2019. Available from: https://www.epocrates.com.

62. Mickan S, Tilson JK, Atherton H, Roberts NW, Heneghan C. Evidence of effectiveness of health care professionals using handheld computers: A scoping review of systematic reviews. *Journal of Medical Internet Research.* 2013;15(10):e212.

63. Johnson E, Emani VK, Ren J. Breadth of coverage, ease of use, and quality of mobile point-of-care tool information summaries: An evaluation. *JMIR mhealth and uhealth.* 2016;4(4):e117.

64. Fjortoft N, Gettig J, Verdone M. Smartphones, memory, and pharmacy education. *American Journal of Pharmaceutical Education.* 2018;82(3):7054.

65. Teodorczuk A, Fraser J, Rogers GD. Open book exams: A potential solution to the "full curriculum"? *Medical Teacher.* 2018;40(5):529–30.

66. Monane M, Matthias DM, Nagle BA, Kelly MA. Improving prescribing patterns for the elderly through an online drug utilization review intervention: A system linking the physician, pharmacist, and computer. *JAMA.* 1998;280(14):1249–52.

67. Muller S. Physicians for the twenty-first century: Report of the project panel on the general professional education of the physician and college preparation for medicine. *Journal of Medical Education.* 1984;59:1–208.

68. Evans RS, Classen DC, Pestotnik SL, Lundsgaarde HP, Burke JP. Improving empiric antibiotic selection using computer decision support. *Archives of Internal Medicine*. 1994;154(8):878–84.

69. Morton CE, Smith SF, Lwin T, George M, Williams M. Computer programming: Should medical students be learning it? *JMIR Medical Education*. 2019;5(1):e11940.

70. Delhi School of Internet Marketing. 30 stats in web marketing you do not know; 2019. Available from: https://dsim.in/blog/2015/07/24/30-stats-in-web-marketing-you-do-not-know/

71. Susskind R, Susskind D. *The Future of the Professions: How Technology Will Transform the Work of Human Experts*. 1st ed. New York: Oxford University Press; 2015:368.

72. Bargiela D, Verkerk MM. The clinician-programmer: Designing the future of medical practice. *The BMJ*. 2013;347:f4563.

73. Kubben PL. Why physicians might want to learn computer programming. *Surgical Neurology International*. 2013;4:30.

74. Mitchell L. *Computing For Medicine: Coding, Data Mining For Med Students*. Toronto: University of Toronto; 2016.

75. McLean A. To code, or not to code. *Canadian Journal of Nursing Informatics*. 2016;11(1). http://tinyurl.com/y3vvg55e

76. Schwab AJ, Wilson SS. Computer literacy in social work. *Computers in Human Services*. 1990;7(1–2):77–92.

77. Fahrni J. Pharmacists should learn to write code; 2013. Available from: https://jerryfahrni.com/page/31/.

78. Matt W. Why every (psychology) student should learn to code. *Computing for Pscyhologists [Internet] 2012*. [06 June 2019]. Available from: https://computingforpsychologists.wordpress.com/2012/01/13/why-every-psychology-student-should-learn-to-code/.

79. AMIA. Clinical Informatics Becomes a Board-certified Medical Subspecialty Following ABMS Vote [press release]. AMIA; 2011. https://www.amia.org/news-and-publications/press-release/ci-is-subspecialty

80. Gardner RM, Overhage JM, Steen EB, Munger BS, Holmes JH, Williamson JJ, et al. Core content for the subspecialty of clinical informatics. *Journal of American Medicine Informatics Association*. 2009;16(2):153–7.

81. World Health Organization. *Framework For Action On Interprofessional Education And Collaborative Practice*. Geneva: World Health Organization; 2010:64.

82. Institute of Medicine. *Measuring the Impact of Interprofessional Education on Collaborative Practice and Patient Outcomes*. Washington, DC: The National Academies Press; 2015.

83. Centre for the Advancement of Interprofessional Education (CAIPE). Statement of purpose: CAIPE; 2016 Available from: https://www.caipe.org/about-us.

84. Murdoch NL, Epp S, Vinek J. Teaching and learning activities to educate nursing students for interprofessional collaboration: A scoping review. *Journal of Interprofessional Care*. 2017;31(6):744–53.

85. Wilhelmsson M, Pelling S, Ludvigsson J, Hammar M, Dahlgren LO, Faresjo T. Twenty years experiences of interprofessional education in Linkoping — ground-breaking and sustainable. *Journal of Interprofessional Care*. 2009;23(2):121–33.

86. Gough S, Hellaby M, Jones N, MacKinnon R. A review of undergraduate interprofessional simulation-based education (IPSE). *Collegian*. 2012;19(3):153–70.

87. Schapmire TJ, Head BA, Nash WA, Yankeelov PA, Furman CD, Wright RB, et al. Overcoming barriers to interprofessional education in gerontology: The interprofessional curriculum for the care of older adults. *Advances in Medical Education and Practice*. 2018;9:109–18.

88. Rogers GD, Thistlethwaite JE, Anderson ES, Abrandt Dahlgren M, Grymonpre RE, Moran M, et al. International consensus statement on the assessment of interprofessional learning outcomes. *Medical Teacher*. 2017;39(4):347–59.

89. Dijamco C. *Staying Sane: Addressing the Growing Concern of Mental Health in Medical Students*. American Medical Student Association; 2015. https://www.amsa.org/2015/09/08/staying-sane-addressing-the-growing-concern-of-mental-health-in-medical-students/

90. Slavin SJ, Schindler DL, Chibnall JT. Medical student mental health 3.0: Improving student wellness through curricular changes. *Academic Medicine*. 2014;89(4):573–7.

91. Kaplan JS, Tolin DF. Exposure therapy for anxiety disorders. *Psychiatric Times*. 2011;28(9): 103–13.

92. Stetz MC, Thomas ML, Russo MB, Stetz TA, Wildzunas RM, McDonald JJ, et al. Stress, mental health, and cognition: a brief review of relationships and countermeasures. *Aviation, Space, and Environmental Medicine*. 2007;78(5 Suppl):B252–60.

93. Flanagan SC, Kotwal RS, Forsten RD. Preparing soldiers for the stress of combat. *Journal of Special Operetaions Medicine*. 2012;12(2):33–41.

94. Manderino MA, Yonkman CA. Stress inoculation: A method of helping students cope with anxiety related to clinical performance. *Journal of Nursing Education*. 1985;24(3):115–8.

95. Chan KD, Humphreys L, Mey A, Holland C, Wu C, Rogers GD. Beyond communication training: the MaRIS model for developing medical students' human capabilities and personal resilience. *Medical Teacher* 2020;42(2):187–95. (DOI: 10.1080/0142159X.2019.1670340)

96. Barbezat DP, Bush M. *Contemplative Practices in Higher Education: Powerful Methods to Transform Teaching and Learning*. 1st ed. California: Jossey-Bass; 2013:256.

97. Wartman SA, Combs CD. Reimagining medical education in the Age of AI. *AMA Journal of Ethics*. 2019;21(2):E146–52.

98. Tversky A, Kahneman D. The framing of decisions and the psychology of choice. *Science*. 1981;211(4481):453–8.

99. de Graaff E, Kolmos, A. *History of Problem-Based and Project-Based Learning. Management of Change: Implementation of Problem-Based and Project-Based Learning in Engineering*. Rotterdam: Brill | Sense; 2007:1–8.

100. Maharg P. The culture of mnemosyne: Open-book assessment and the theory and practice of legal education. *International Journal of the Legal Profession*. 1999;6(2):219–39.

101. Harden RM, Gleeson FA. Assessment of clinical competence using an objective structured clinical examination (OSCE). *Medical Education*. 1979;13(1):41–54.

102. Norcini JJ, Blank LL, Arnold GK, Kimball HR. The mini-CEX (clinical evaluation exercise): A preliminary investigation. *Annals of Internal Medicine*. 1995;123(10):795–9.

103. Kotter JP. Leading change: Why transformation efforts fail. *Harvard Business Review*. 1995; March–April:59–67.

104. Wartman SA. *Medicine and Machines: The Coming Transformation of Healthcare*. Washington, DC: Association of Academic Health Centers; 2016.

105. Hernán-Losada I, Velázquez-Iturbide JÁ, Lázaro C. Programming learning tools based on Bloom's taxonomy: Proposal and accomplishments. *Proceedings of the 8th International Symposium of Computers in Education (SIIE 2006)*. (Leon, Spain, October 24-26). 2006:343–51.

106. Johnson CG, Fuller U. Is Bloom's taxonomy appropriate for computer science? *Proceedings of the 6th Baltic Sea conference on Computing Education Research, Koli Calling; 2006; Uppsala, Sweden*. 1315825: ACM; 2006:120–3.

107. Lahtinen E. A Categorization of novice programmers: A cluster analysis study. PPIG 2007 — 19th Annual Workshop; 2007.

108. Fuller U, Johnson CG, Ahoniemi T, Cukierman D, Hernán-Losada I, Jackova J, et al. Developing a computer science-specific learning taxonomy. *ACM SIGCSE Bulletin*. 2007;39(4):152–70.

109. Rigby MJ. From the editor: Ethical dimensions of using artificial intelligence in health care. *AMA Journal of Ethics*. 2019;21(2):e121–4.

110. Shortliffe EH. Biomedical informatics in the education of physicians. *JAMA*. 2010;304(11): 1227–8.

111. Sanchez-Mendiola M, Martinez-Franco AI, Lobato-Valverde M, Fernandez-Saldivar F, Vives-Varela T, Martinez-Gonzalez A. Evaluation of a biomedical informatics course for medical students: A pre-posttest study at UNAM faculty of medicine in Mexico. *BMC Medical Education*. 2015;15:64.

112. Teng T, Wu D, Wang G. Using Information technology to integrate Pathology Course and Information Literacy as Part of Instruction. 2016 8th International Conference on Information Technology in Medicine and Education (ITME), Los Alamitos CA: *IEEE Computer Society*. 2016:840–3.

113. Silverman H, Cohen T, Fridsma D. The evolution of a novel biomedical informatics curriculum for medical students. *Academic Medicine*. 2012;87(1):84–90.

114. Combes B. Generation Y. Are they really digital natives or more like digital refugees? *Synergy*. 2009;7(1):31–40.

115. Baker J. Coding to be mandatory in primary, early high school. *The Sydney Morning Herald*; 2018. Available from: https://www.smh.com.au/national/nsw/coding-to-be-mandatory-in-primary-early-high-school-20180817-p4zy5d.html

116. Rogers GD, Parker-Tomlin M, Clanchy K, Townshend J, Chan P. C. Utilising a post-placement critical assessment task to consolidate interprofessional learning. In: S. Billett JN, G. D. Rogers, C. Noble, editors. *Augmenting Health and Social Care Students' Clinical Learning Experiences*. Dordrecht, Germany: Springer; 2019:73–94.

117. Rogers GD, McConnell HW, de Rooy NJ, Ellem F, Lombard M. A randomised controlled trial of extended immersion in multi-method continuing simulation to prepare senior medical students for practice as junior doctors. *BMC Medical Education*. 2014;14:90.

118. Rogers GD, Mey A, Chan PC. Development of a phenomenologically derived method to assess affective learning in student journals following impactive educational experiences. *Medical Teacher*. 2017;39(12):1250–60.

119. Seefeldt TM, Mort JR, Brockevelt B, Giger J, Jordre B, Lawler M, et al. A pilot study of interprofessional case discussions for health professions students using the virtual world Second Life. *Currents in Pharmacy Teaching and Learning*. 2012;4(4):224–31.

120. Davis D, Hercelinskyj G, Jackson L. Promoting interprofessional collaboration: A pilot project using simulation in the virtual world of second life. *Journal of Research in Interprofessional Practice and Education*. 2016;6(2):E1–E15.

121. Reed B (Editor). (1974). Star trek: The animated series. [TV series episode]. In: L. Scheimer (Producer). *The Practical Joker*. New York: National Broadcasting Company.

122. Zhu E, Hadadgar A, Masiello I, Zary N. Augmented reality in healthcare education: An integrative review. *PeerJ*. 2014;2:e469.

123. McCallum, R. (Producer) & Lucas, G. (Director). (1999). *Star Wars Episode I — The Phantom Menace* [Motion picture]. USA: Lucasfilm Ltd.

124. Shapiro SL, Schwartz GE, Bonner G. Effects of mindfulness-based stress reduction on medical and premedical students. *Journal of Behavioral Medicine*. 1998;21(6):581–99.

125. Rogers G, Mey A, Chan P, Lombard M, Miller F. Development and validation of the Griffith University affective learning scale (GUALS): A tool for assessing affective learning in health professional students' reflective journals. *MedEdPublish*. 2018;7(1):1–13.

126. Dietschie E. Google Glass gains headway in healthcare. *MedCityNews*. 2017. https://medcitynews.com/2017/07/google-glass-healthcare/?rf=1.

127. NSW Agency for Clinical Innovation. *Understanding and Working with General Practice*. New South Wales, Australia: NSW Agency for Clinical Innovation; 2015.

128. Ayatollahi A, Ayatollahi J, Ayatollahi F, Ayatollahi R, Shahcheraghi SH. Computer and internet use among undergraduate medical students in Iran. *Pakistan Journal Medical Sciences*. 2014;30(5):1054–8.

129. Sulzenbruck S, Hegele M, Rinkenauer G, Heuer H. The death of handwriting: Secondary effects of frequent computer use on basic motor skills. *Journal Motor Behavior*. 2011;43(3):247–51.

130. ExamSoft. ExamSoft. Available from: https://examsoft.com/.

131. Mathew H. Transforming Exams: Processes and platform for e-Exams in supervised BYOD environments: Australian Government office for learning and teaching; 2019. Available from: https://ltr.edu.au/resources/SD13_2885_Hillier_Report_2014.pdf

132. Frohna JG, Gruppen LD, Fliegel JE, Mangrulkar RS. Development of an evaluation of medical student competence in evidence-based medicine using a computer-based OSCE station. *Teaching and Learning in Medicine*. 2006;18(3):267–72.

133. Fraser SW, Greenhalgh T. Coping with complexity: Educating for capability. *The BMJ*. 2001;323(7316):799–803.

INDEX

CPSIA information can be obtained
at www.ICGtesting.com
Printed in the USA
FSHW021632160421
80458FS